# CANCER

of the

# URINARY BLADDER

*A Monograph in*

MODERN CONCEPTS OF RADIOLOGY,
NUCLEAR MEDICINE AND ULTRASOUND

*Series Editor*

LEWIS E. ETTER, M.D., F.A.C.R.

*Professor of Radiology*
*Western Psychiatric Institute and Falk Clinic*
*Presbyterian-University Hospital*
*School of Medicine*
*University of Pittsburgh*
*Pittsburgh, Pennsylvania*

# CANCER

## of the

# URINARY BLADDER

*With Emphasis on Treatment by Irradiation*

*By*

## WILLIAM L. CALDWELL, M.D.

*Professor of Radiology*
*Director of Radiotherapy and Radiation Research*
*Vanderbilt University Hospital*
*Nashville, Tennessee*

WARREN H. GREEN, INC.
*St. Louis, Missouri, U.S.A.*

*Published by*

WARREN H. GREEN, INC.
10 South Brentwood Blvd.
St. Louis, Missouri 63105, U.S.A.

*Library of Congress Catalog Card No. 72-96980*

*Printed in the United States of America*
2-A                                            150

*This monograph is dedicated to my wife, Theron,
and my children: Ben, Sam, Alan, Megan, Erica, and Bret
of whom I am so proud*

# Preface

THE field of oncology spans a breadth of specialties, specialties in which some involved physicians spend only a small percentage of their time managing patients with cancer. Hence, their individual experience with the treatment of cancer may be limited. Furthermore, such physicians often are not totally aware of the various treatment methods which might be best suited for their particular patient. Consultation and advice from others may be warranted. In urologic oncology, in particular, consultation between urologist and radiotherapist almost always is mutually beneficial and of undeniable importance to the patient.

In this monograph on treatment of *Cancer of the Bladder,* an effort has been made to present a guide for those treating patients with bladder cancer. Present knowledge as to epidemiology, etiology, and natural history is reviewed. Then, following discussions of clinical evaluation, histologic grading and staging, various radiotherapeutic, operative and chemotherapeutic approaches to management are considered. Results of current treatment by various methods are tabulated. Meaningful comparison of results between different treatment methods is thwarted by the lack of similarity between patients included in the series. Differences in staging, result reporting, and other factors make valid and definite conclusions regarding therapy impossible. Yet, there are clues from the review. They are incorporated in the ideas expressed in the final chapter, entitled "Treatment Recommendations."

It is hoped that sufficient questions and controversy will be stimulated to provide an impetus for initiation of a comprehensive, randomized study of the treatment of bladder cancer by various methods among many cooperating institutions. Such a study should provide better data to help establish the most effective current therapy for controlling different stages and types of bladder cancer, with suitable attention given to morbidity and mortality associated with such treatment.

# Acknowledgments

SINCERE appreciation is extended to Mrs. Elizabeth Shipp, Mrs. Evelyn Sexton, Miss Barbara Burr, Mrs. Betty Angevine, and Mrs. Karen Aristizabal for secretarial assistance and for their patience with me during my seemingly endless redrafts.

Mr. Colin Woodham, radiation physicist at the Division of Radiotherapy, Vanderbilt University Hospital, kindly provided the majority of figures used, including all the radiotherapy plans in Chapter 6. Dr. H. J. G. Bloom supplied several figures used in Chapter 6. Dr. J. F. Fraumeni, Jr. provided 2 figures included in Chapter 2. To these individuals I am most appreciative.

The author has profited greatly by review of the experience, wisdom, and thoughts of the many authors who have made significant contributions regarding bladder cancer to the medical literature. The quotations of some of these contributors are included in this monograph because of their unusual merits of content and clarity of presentation.

Mr. Warren H. Green, publisher, and Dr. Lewis E. Etter, editor, gave significant counsel and encouragement during preparation. Without this assistance the whole project might have faltered.

Also my appreciation to the patience of my understanding wife and children of my prolonged absences or periods of inattention during the preparation of this monograph.

W.L.C.

# Contents

# CANCER

of the

# URINARY BLADDER

*Chapter 1*

# Introduction: The Bladder Cancer Problem

P AST cancer mortality statistics predicted that approximately 8,500 persons in the United States were expected to die from cancer of the urinary bladder in 1968;[88] this represents about 3.5 per cent of all cancer deaths. Furthermore, statistics show that the mortality rate from this cause is increasing slightly, not only in the United States but in other countries as well. This is particularly so in industrial centers. One of the highest mortality rates for bladder neoplasms has been in England and Wales, with an annual death rate of 6.8 per 100,000 males, and the lowest mortality in Japan, with 1.9 per 100,000; the annual death rate in this country is intermediate with 5.2 per 100,000.[104]

The true incidence of malignant neoplasms of the urinary bladder in the United States is uncertain since cancer is not a reportable disease in most states. Nevertheless, because no fewer than 70-75 per cent of *all* patients with carcinoma of the bladder die with disease, it can be estimated that approximately 12,000-14,000 new cases of bladder malignancy are discovered each year in this country.[104, 154, 299, 300]

Cancer of the urinary bladder is more frequent in males than females by a ratio of approximately 3:1 and is responsible for about 4.5 per cent of all deaths secondary to malignancy in males, and for about 1.5 per cent of all cancer deaths in females.[273, 299] It is a disease of old age, with a sharp increase in incidence in the late 6th and early 7th decades.[299] However, a greater number of cases have been seen in recent years in younger age groups. The reason for this is uncertain.

In the United States, carcinoma of the urinary bladder is more common in whites than non-whites for males; however, this difference is declining. The incidence of urinary bladder cancer in females is similar for whites and non-whites.[299]

There is no clearly established difference of religious preference, degree of education, place of residence, amount of liquid intake, or the degree of alcohol intake between patients with malignant disease of the urinary bladder and matched controls. Tumors of the urinary bladder are seen more frequently in single persons or those not currently married, particularly among divorced males; the reason for this is not certain. An apparent increased risk of bladder cancer is documented for tobacco users, for persons with chronic bladder infections, retention, or calculi, and for industrial workers involved in the use of certain chemicals; this will be detailed in a subsequent chapter.[154, 299, 300]

No strong familial link for neoplasms of the bladder has been observed. Multiple cases within a family have been reported; Fraumeni and Thomas,[103] e.g., recently have seen carcinoma of the urinary bladder in a father and three of his sons. Nevertheless, such occurrences are rare.

Other epidemiologic aspects of bladder cancers presumably will be noted in the future. This may allow for earlier detection in high risk patients with resultant improvement in survival probabilities.

# Chapter 2

# Etiology

THERE is considerable knowledge about the etiology of bladder neoplasms, at least some bladder neoplasms. Bladder tumors occur frequently in chemical, rubber, and cable workers, individuals who are exposed to antioxidants, solvents, or other carcinogens.[49, 67, 71, 222, 276] Exposure may be from either skin contact or from the vapor. The risk probably is related to the degree of exposure to these agents. Hairdressers, gas retort house workers, shoe leather workers, textile dye workers, painters, and others also have been shown to be at greater risks than the population at large.[49, 64, 66, 67, 134, 154, 183, 214, 257, 273, 276, 299, 300]

In 1895, Rehn[231] reported that at least 3, and perhaps 4, workers in a group of 45 men producing fuchsin were found to have bladder tumors; rightly this was considered more than a coincidence for such an uncommon tumor. Aniline vapor was suggested by Rehn as being the likely offender since fuchsin was made by the oxidation of aniline. Impurities in the aniline were considered contributors to the carcinogenesis as well. Recent studies indicate that aniline itself probably is not carcinogenic, but confirm that intermediate agents used in the manufacture of fuchsin, as well as auramine, undoubtedly are.[28]

*five*

B-naphthylamine was suggested by Leichtenstern in 1898 as a possible bladder carcinogen in man and it indeed has been proven a potent carcinogen. In 1938, Hueper[135] induced bladder tumors in dogs by oral administration of commercial B-naphthylamine. Scott and Boyd[247] and others[237, 246] later confirmed these results. Benzidine and a-naphthylamine also were found to be definite occupational hazards, as were 4-aminodiphenyl (xenylamine) and 4-nitrodiphenyl;[190] the aromatic amines are excreted as orthohydroxylated urinary metabolites. Experimental bladder tumors now also have been induced by polycyclic hydrocarbons, a variety of aromatic amines, and other non-nitrogenous compounds.[229, 237] Hueper[134] has shown that 2-amino-1-naphthol is locally carcinogenic when injected into the mouse. Forty-five to 50 per cent of hamsters fed a diet containing 0.1 per cent o-amino azotoluene will develop urinary bladder cancer in 49 weeks.[261]

During the years 1902 to 1958, exposure to B-naphthylamine and benzidine resulted in at least 350 cases of bladder cancer in Germany. Approximately 80,000 cases of fatal "spontaneous" bladder cancer of the male population were reported during the same period of time.[257]

Recently, the hazard of bladder cancer induction in rubber industry workers was evaluated by Case.[49] A significantly increased risk was shown (Table 2-I), particularly in those working in Birmingham County Borough.

Case[49] also studied 4,622 men who were employed by one of the 21 member firms of the Association of British Chemical Manufacturers. All persons included had been employed by one of the participating companies for at least 6 months during the 1910 to 1952 period. Three to five deaths from bladder tumors would have been anticipated in this group. The observed number of deaths was 127, approximately 30 times as great as predicted. The average latent period between the time of initial exposure and diagnosis of a tumor was 18 years, varying from 5 to 45 years. Oppenheimer[214] found a similar average with a range of 8 to 41 years; Poole-Wilson[221] found an average latent period of 20.5 years.

A cohort study of 639 males employed in 1938 or 1939 in an

*six*

TABLE 2-I

NUMBER OF DEATH CERTIFICATES WHERE TUMOR OF THE BLADDER
WAS MENTIONED RELATING TO WORKERS* IN RUBBER
OCCUPATIONS, BIRMINGHAM COUNTY BOROUGH AND ENGLAND
AND WALES, 1952-1961 (MODIFIED FROM CASE)[49]

|  | 1952-1956 | 1957-1961 |
|---|---|---|
| Birmingham County Borough |  |  |
| Observed | 10 | 12 |
| Expected | 1.3 | 1.5 |
| England and Wales, except |  |  |
| Birmingham County Borough |  |  |
| Observed | 10 | 15 |
| Expected | 8.5 | 9.5 |

* Includes men who at the time of death were either occupied or retired.

American company manufacturing B-naphthylamine and benzidine followed to 1965 was conducted by Manusco and El-
Attar.[183] Malignancy of the bladder and kidney constituted 35
per cent of all malignant neoplasms occurring in these individuals. The observed mortality rate for cancer of the bladder
for white men (26 to 65 years of age) was 78/100,000 in the
cohort as compared with 4.4/100,000 for white Ohio men of
those ages. For "exposed" employees, the rate was 335/100,000
for ages 45 to 64 years and 971/100,000 for ages 65 or over.
Hueper[134] estimates that well over 500 cases of occupational
bladder cancer have been diagnosed among American chemical
workers. Although there is no effective legislation in the United
States (except in the State of Pennsylvania) for the regulation
of use, manufacture, and importation of proven carcinogenic
solvents and other chemicals, these are no longer in use by most
industries. Substitutes have proven less hazardous. Nevertheless,
the incidence of bladder cancer, particularly in industrial com-
munities, continues to rise.

The pathogenesis of chemically induced bladder tumors apparently is similar to those occurring spontaneously. During
the latent interval, the bladder epithelium is not normal; in
fact, exfoliated cells may be abnormal for months or years before the clinical recognition of a tumor. The same phenomenon
has been demonstrated in beagle dogs by Deichman[71] with tran-

sition of mucosal pattern from normal, to pre-neoplastic, to pre-cancerous, to cancerous. In the three major high risk industries in England, urinary cytology screening is being applied as a routine, regularly scheduled measure in all employees, in an effort to detect early mucosal abnormalities.[276] The value of this technique will be discussed under diagnosis.

Numerous reviews on industrial bladder cancer are in the recent literature;[24, 66, 67] several include exhaustive bibliographies. A symposium on the occupational aspects of bladder cancer, held at the Fifth Inter-American Conference on Toxicology and Occupational Medicine, was published in 1967;[71,] the available knowledge on incidence and etiology of bladder cancer of industrial origin is summarized. *Industrial and Experimental Bladder Cancer,* by Price,[222] published in 1966, summarizes the present status of the title problem; a comprehensive literature listing is provided.

Because tryptophan metabolites resemble chemically known bladder carcinogens, altered tryptophan metabolism has been thought a likely cause for spontaneous bladder tumor. There is one species of animal, the cat, which appears to be immune to bladder cancer. A study of the tryptophan metabolism of this animal by Price[222] has shown that the cat metabolizes tryptophan to amino-hippuric acid and not to kynurenine or anthanalic acid as occurs in man, the dog, and other experimental animals. Some patients with bladder tumors have high urinary concentrations of tryptophan breakdown products, excreting substantially more kynurenine, kynurenic acid, and acetyl kynurenine than normal subjects. Efforts to isolate a definite carcinogenic breakdown product, however, have not been successful.

Eight out of ten rats given 2-acetamidofluorene in a diet in which the protein was replaced by an acid casein hydrolysate and 2 per cent dl-tryptophan developed tumors of the urinary bladder;[30] ordinarily 2-acetamidofluorene and a high protein diet will cause liver and ear cancers. Perhaps the combination of 2-acetamidofluorene and tryptophan metabolites results in a summation of carcinogenic stimuli. Because pyridoxine can nearly always reduce the level of urinary tryptophan metabo-

*eight*

lites in both health and disease, it has received attention as a potential inhibitor of bladder carcinogenesis. Evidence of its clinical effectiveness, however, is still lacking.

Boyland[29] has attempted to provide prophylaxis of bladder cancer by oral administration of an ammonium salt of $1 \rightarrow 4$-glucosaccharolactone, a potent inhibitor of B-glucuronidase. Glucosiduronic acids are hydrolyzed by B-glucuronidase into presumed active metabolites. One hundred and three cases included in their study had Stage A carcinoma of the bladder, treated by diathermy alone; all were free of tumor at cystoscopy at the start of the trial. Recurrence rates were similar in patients given $1 \rightarrow 4$-glucosaccharolactone (4 gm qd), lactose (8 gm qd), or sodium potassium citrate tablets (6 gms qd for alkalinization).

An increase in urinary tryptophan metabolites has been reported in smokers,[52] and according to some reports, cigarette smoking is associated with an increased risk of developing bladder tumor. Deeley and Cohen[70] noted that only 3 out of 127 of their patients with carcinoma of the bladder had never smoked as compared with 9 out of 127 of a matched control group. Patients with carcinoma of the bladder had, on an average,

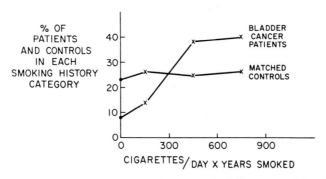

SMOKING HISTORY OF 163
PATIENTS WITH BLADDER CANCER
(MODIFIED FROM YOSHIDA)

FIGURE 2-1. The proportion of individuals with different smoking histories is compared in patients with bladder cancer and in matched controls. A significant relationship is demonstrated, the bladder cancer patients tending to be much heavier smokers than the controls.

*nine*

smoked more than control patients as well. In a series of patients studied at the Veterans Administration in Seattle, Cobb and Ansell[52] noted that 104 of 131 patients with carcinoma of the bladder were heavy tobacco users, whereas only 52 of 120 patients in a control group with carcinoma of the colon were heavy smokers. Lockwood,[170] likewise, demonstrated a statistical association between excessive tobacco consumption and benign and malignant bladder tumors. Figure 2-1 indicates the effect of degree of smoking on the incidence of cancer of the bladder, according to Yoshida.[300]

Compilation of results from 7 studies evaluating the effect of smoking on the incidence of bladder cancer is shown in Table 2-II.[154] Ex-smokers apparently do not carry the increase in risk they had when smoking. Also shown in the same table is the finding by Doll[77] in a prospective study involving a large group of British physicians whose smoking habits were known and well documented; this is one of two reported series showing no apparent relationship between smoking and bladder cancer. Similarly, statistical evaluation of lung and bladder cancer deaths among the inhabitants of 163 American metropolitan areas clearly demonstrates that the remarkable discrepancies in lung and bladder cancer rates observed militate strongly against a single causal factor, such as cigarette smoking, for both neoplasms. "A comparison between cities with high and low lung cancer rates and high and low bladder cancer rates reveals such a lack of parallelism between the cancer rates for both organs that cigarette smoking can be excluded as a major factor in the production of bladder cancers among the inhabitants of the United States," states Heuper.[134] However, a recent report by

TABLE 2-II

RELATIVE RISK OF CANCER OF THE BLADDERS FOR SMOKERS
(ADAPTED FROM KING AND BAILER)[154]

| Study Group | Expected Deaths | Observed Deaths | Mortality Rates |
|---|---|---|---|
| Cigarette Smokers | 111.6 | 216 | 1.9 |
| Ex-cigarette Smokers | 29.8 | 31 | 1.0 |
| British Doctors, Cigarette Smokers | 13.9 | 12 | 0.9 |

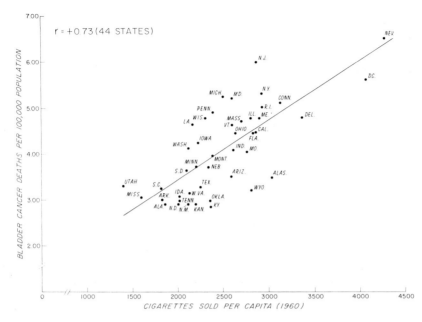

FIGURE 2-2. The relationship between bladder cancer mortality and per capita cigarette sales in 44 states is demonstrated.[102]

Fraumeni[102] demonstrates a high correlation between per capita cigarette sales and bladder cancer mortality rates in 44 states of the United States; Figure 2-2 depicts this. The correlation is almost identical to that seen between per capita cigarette sales and lung cancer mortality; this relationship is shown in Figure 2-3. The explanation for the sharp differences between these studies, all by competent epidemiologists and statisticians, is not apparent.

Kerr[153] has shown that toxic aminophenols occur in excessive amounts in the urine of smokers; a metabolic block is suggested to explain this. Cobb and Ansell[52] noted that enzymes in the bladder hydrolyze the tobacco breakdown products, glucosiduronic acid or a sulfuric ester, resulting in the release of an active agent. This explains the specificity of the compounds for the bladder rather than for the ureter or kidney pelvis. Such a concept for pathogenesis would be consistent with the observation that bladder neck obstruction is associated with a high incidence of bladder cancers; neoplasms also are frequent in di-

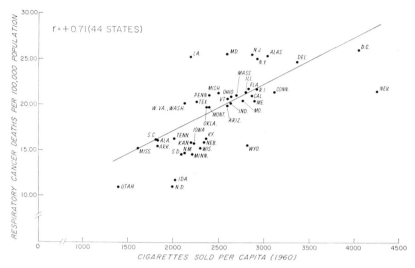

FIGURE 2-3. A similar (to Fig. 2-2) relationship is shown for lung cancer mortality.[102]

verticula, another situation where urine stasis is encountered.[23] Nineteen (7 per cent) of 285 consecutive cases of vesical diverticulum reported by McLean and Kelalis[178] contained malignant lesions. Most were infiltrating and a third were squamous cell carcinomas. Stasis was present in 20 per cent of all male cases of urinary bladder tumors seen by Wallace.[273]

Holsti and Ermala[132] have produced papillary carcinomas of the bladder in adult "albino mice of a mixed known strain" after per oral administration of tobacco tars. The oral cavity of mice had been swabbed daily with tobacco tar in an effort to cause oral cavity tumors at routine autopsy, an unexpected finding was papillary carcinoma of the urinary bladder in 15 per cent of the animals who survived. Benign papillomatosis occurred in 87.5 per cent of the animals. No spontaneous tumors occur in this strain under usual circumstances. Chapman[51] was unable to confirm these effects in male BALB/c mice.

Carcinoma of the bladder also has been seen frequently in patients with severe infestation with Schistosoma hematobium.[113, 180, 208] Bladder calcification, a sign of severe and chronic infestation, is noted more frequently in bladder cancer patients

*twelve*

than in controls.[113] Ova deposition in the rectum also is seen more often and is more severe when present in the bladder cancer patients. These tumors tend to develop in a relatively younger age group than does carcinoma of the bladder from other causes; 69 per cent of the patients reported by Gelfand and associates[113] in patients with severe chronic bilharzial disease of the bladder were under the age of 50 years. Another interesting finding is that the majority of tumors associated with bilharzial infestation are of the squamous cell type.

Bovine urinary bladder tumors have been endemic to certain parts of the world such as Turkey, Yugoslavia, Bulgaria, Panama, and Brazil.[216] Virus induced transitional cell carcinomas of the bladder have been produced in cows.[37] Recently, bracken fern (Pteris aquilina) was fed to 18 cows by Pamukcu and associates.[216] Ten of the eighteen animals developed neoplasms of the urinary bladder, and 3 of these lesions were carcinomas. Two of the carcinomas invaded the muscle wall of the bladder and were found $2\frac{1}{2}$ to $3\frac{1}{2}$ years after initiation of feeding. The carcinogenic substance in bracken fern has not as yet been identified.

Clearly, numerous noxious agents are capable of inducing bladder tumors. Nevertheless, fewer than 3 per cent of all human bladder tumors are due to a suspected etiologic agent. Possibly small quantities of currently unrecognized chemicals may be implicated ultimately. With forebearance and perseverance other specific causative agents may be discovered. While new carcinogens are being found, every effort must be made to restrict exposure to known carcinogenic agents.

## Chapter 3

# Diagnosis and Pretreatment Evaluation

THE most common pretreatment signs and symptoms of bladder malignancy include hematuria (in as many as 95 per cent of patients), increase in frequency, and urodynia. Hematuria characteristically is intermittent, often a factor in delay in establishing a diagnosis.[165] Hematuria, of course, is always an alarming sign; it should trigger an exhaustive investigative search for a cause. Pain is a late symptom and indicates a poor prognosis. Loss of weight is a very late symptom and is associated with a virtually hopeless prognosis.[260] Obstruction is a frequent presenting complaint in the childhood sarcomas.

Physical examination may yield evidence of metastatic disease either in peripheral lymph nodes, the liver, or bones. A pelvic mass may be palpable through the abdominal wall or on bimanual examination in a female. The prostate should be examined for evidence of involvement in males.

Laboratory studies should include a white blood cell count, a hematocrit, urinalysis and urine culture, particularly if there is increased frequency and urodynia. Either a blood urea nitrogen or serum creatinine level also should be obtained. An alka-

*fourteen*

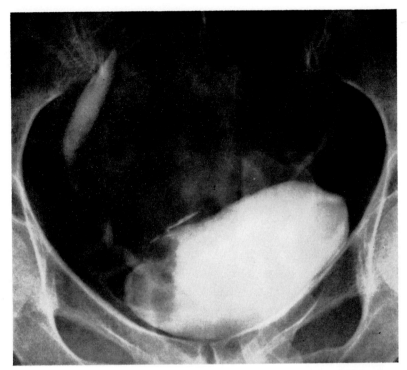

FIGURE 3-1. Delayed film of an excretory urogram clearly delineating a papillary tumor on the right lateral wall of the bladder. There is a partial obstruction of the right urethral orifice with proximal dilation of the right ureter.

line phosphatase determination can exclude the presence of gross hepatic or osseous metastases.

Radiologic investigation should include a chest x-ray and a radiographic bone survey, particularly if there are osseous symptoms. An excretory urogram may demonstrate evidence of ureteral obstruction or disease in the upper urinary tract. The bladder tumor itself may be seen with delayed films of the bladder (Fig. 3-1),[4] but rarely does this demonstrate the tumor as well as double or triple contrast cystograms (Figs. 3-2 and 3-3).[78, 161, 258]

Doyle[78, 79] and Glanville[115] have shown the value of single and double contrast cystography using 100 to 150 milliliters of Steripaque® (sterilized suspension of barium sulfate) initially.

*fifteen*

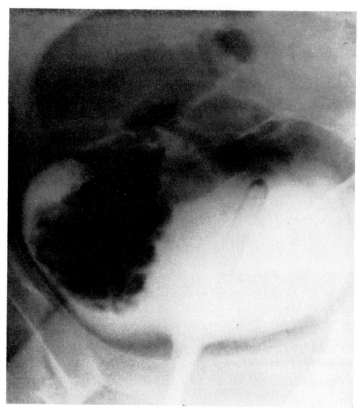

FIGURE 3-2. A papillary bladder tumor along the lateral wall of the bladder is shown by single contrast (Renografin® in the bladder) technique.

After the necessary films are exposed, all but 20 to 30 milliliters of the barium suspension is removed and the bladder is then distended with either nitrous oxide or carbon dioxide. Site, size, and multiplicity of tumors may be ascertained on subsequent radiographs. The width of the tumor base may influence therapy; malignant tumors have broader bases than papillomas. Bladder wall infiltration causes an irregular outline and a rigidity of the wall with lack of normal distensibility. Pseudo diverticular formation also indicates infiltration; Doyle[79] has shown with a bladder analogue the mechanisms for this. Ureteral reflux is occasionally seen and until explained otherwise is considered evidence for infiltration around the ureteral orifice.

Displacement of the bladder means spread outside of the bladder. Fixation of the bladder is not readily established and muscular infiltration alone can cause apparent fixation radiographically.

Connolly and associates[57] have found fractionated cystograms useful in distinguishing between superficial and infiltrating tumors of the bladder. A constant amount of iodinated contrast material is instilled through a catheter in each of four increments, the total volume equalling the bladder capacity. After each increment of contrast medium is instilled, with the patient remaining immobile between instillations, superimposed exposures are made in 4 projections (anterior-posterior with 10 degree tilt toward the patient's feet, lateral, and both obliques), a single film being used for each of the 4 views. At sites of

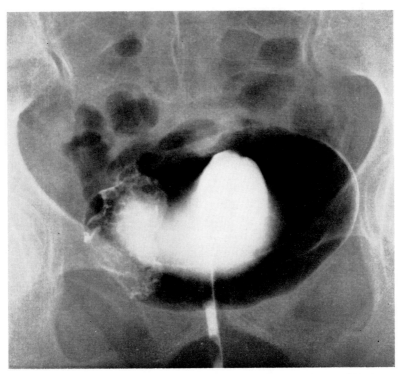

FIGURE 3-3. Double contrast (Renografin® and $CO_2$ in the bladder) exam also demonstrates a right lateral wall papillary bladder tumor.

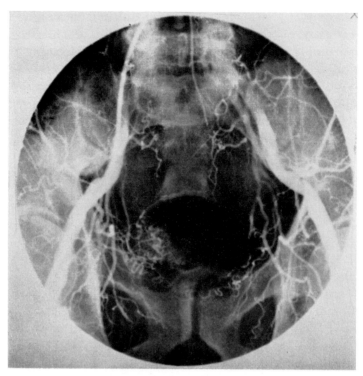

FIGURE 3-4A. Tumor vascularity in the base of the bladder on the right ($CO_2$ in the bladder for contrast).

muscular infiltration, no distention can be demonstrated as the bladder expands.

To better demonstrate or diagnose suspected extravesical spread, injection of the perivesical space with 200 to 300 milliliters of carbon dioxide will provide a clear demonstration of the bladder wall thickness, except at the base.[12] Selective angiography, with or without perivesical gas insufflation, also may provide useful information (Figs. 3-4A and 4B) regarding the extent of the tumor.[22, 151, 160, 161, 213, 295] Often unexpected local extension is demonstrated.

Lang[161] has succinctly reviewed the technique in a recent article. A Seldinger catheter is introduced into the femoral artery and advanced to the level of the bifurcation. After injection of iodinated contrast material through the catheter, serial radiographs are taken over a period from 0 to 14 seconds. Films may be taken in multiple projections to better define the tumor and the depth of infiltration. Abnormal vessels may be seen extending through the muscular wall into the perivesical spaces. "Corkscrew" vessels, arteriovenous lakes, and an early venous return phase are characteristic of anaplastic tumors. A dense tumor stain is more frequently seen in low grade tumors. Abnormal vessels and arterio-venous shunts are not seen in inflammatory conditions and the presence of these abnormalities establishes the diagnosis of cancer. The bladder normally receives virtually all of its blood from branches of the internal-iliac artery—the superior vesical, inferior vesical, and mid vesical arteries. Minor contributions from the pudendal and obtu-

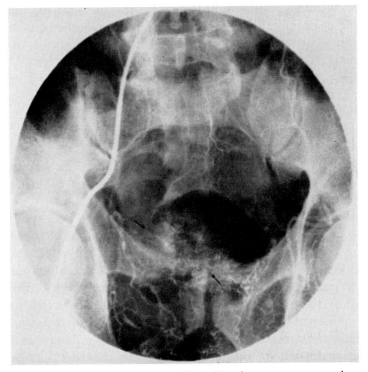

FIGURE 3-4B. Tumor stain on delayed film. Vessels appear to extend outside of wall of the bladder suggesting it is a Stage C tumor, or possibly a Stage D tumor. Perivesical insufflation might have been helpful.

*nineteen*

rator arteries may be seen. Supply by an extraneous vascular system is considered a definite evidence of invasion outside the perivesical space and therefore is sufficient evidence for a Stage D classification.

The triple contrast cystograms in conjunction with selective arteriography have a 84 per cent accuracy rate in pathologic Stage $B_2$ and C tumors. Tumors tend to be overstaged (as compared to the pathologic stage) more frequently by this method whereas, of course, other clinical methods consistently understage lesions.[161]

These angiographic studies, in particular, are difficult and time consuming examinations, and therefore are expensive. Presently they are the most accurate means of clinically staging urinary bladder tumors. However, at this time, these diagnostic studies are used routinely in so few institutions that the findings on these examinations should perhaps not influence clinical staging. If investigators do use these studies in clinically staging some or all patients, then their patients should be staged both with and without the benefit of the radiographic findings on these examinations.

Lymphangiography is used rarely, if at all, in most institutions. Occasionally, definite lymph node metastases may be demonstrated. However, criteria for definitely diagnosing small foci in lymph nodes have not been established. The findings on this examination should not currently be considered in clinical staging of patients.

A definite diagnosis will be established only by cystoscopy.[5] The position, extent, and nature of the tumor must be evaluated carefully. The tumor should be described adequately as being either papillary or solid, ulcerated or non-ulcerated, sessile or pedunculated. The status of the surrounding mucosa is noted; is there leukoplakia, hypertrophy, chronic cystitis, etc.? The presence of obstruction, trabeculation, diverticula, and prostatic enlargement or involvement should be determined. Often, it is difficult cystoscopically to differentiate between benign and malignant papillary growths; in some instances there may be co-existent benign and malignant tumors in the same bladder. Several representative specimens should be obtained with the resectoscope for histologic evaluation. The depth of the lesions

*twenty*

should be biopsied so as to determine the degree of bladder wall penetration; the biopsies are ordinarily best obtained from the margin, particularly if the lesion is ulcerated, although the depth of penetration may be misleading if the lesion is large. Biopsies lateral to the tumor may demonstrate circumferential spread of the cancer not suspected by endoscopic appearance. An adequate biopsy permits assessment of the histologic pattern, grade of tumor, presence of lymphatic permeation and the depth of penetration into the bladder wall. This information is important in determining the type of therapy necessary.

Jewett[141] has described the biopsy process precisely. The important steps involve: "1) placing in bottle 1 all the pieces of that part of the tumor which projects into the cavity of the bladder, a step which takes resection down to the level of the surrounding bladder mucosa, and 2) placing in bottle 2 all the pieces that one scoops out of the bladder muscle beneath the tumor, usually to the depth of 1 loop. It is dangerous to go deeper than this in the upper portions of the bladder, but in the lower, fixed portion, a third layer of thin slivers can be taken if necessary. The pathologist should be notified of the significance of the different bottles and especially that the deep side of each fragment will have a convex contour corresponding to the shape of the loop." With biopsy specimens carefully taken in this way and properly sectioned, unsuspected deep infiltration will be present only rarely. Close cooperation with the pathologist allows the preliminary clinical assessment to coincide with the pathologic findings in as many as 75 per cent of cases.[273]

With open biopsy, Milner[200] has suggested that it should be transfixed vertically with a common pin before sending it to the laboratory. The pathologist may then be able to imbed it in the paraffin block in such a way as to make vertical sections possible.

Adequate specimens are essential; otherwise the most malignant portion of the tumor may not be examined histologically.[235] Dean[68] compared the malignancy of bladder tumors as shown by cystoscopic biopsy to that after examination of the entire bladder. The grade of malignancy was found to be the same in 42 per cent. Examination of the bladder showed tumor

*twenty-one*

of a higher grade of malignancy in 50 per cent. In 4 per cent, the cystoscopic biopsy showed tumor of a higher grade of malignancy than examination of the entire bladder. In 4 per cent of the instances, there were multiple cystoscopic biopsies which showed different grades of malignancy. Franksson[101] found differences in histological grade in different portions of large biopsy specimens of bladder tumor in 72 of 132 cases.

Cystoscopic examinations should be done under general anesthesia to allow bimanual examination of the pelvis with the patient satisfactorily relaxed. Wallace[273] has stressed the importance of this procedure and has listed common mistakes committed during bimanual examination. "Inadequate relaxation and a full bladder make evaluation difficult. If the tumor is at the fundus, it may be missed because digital pressure above the symphysis directed downward and backward towards the rectum may displace the tumor upward towards the umbilicus; the abdominal fingers should always start near the umbilicus and move down towards the symphysis. In cases with palpable fundal tumors, the neoplasm will be felt to slip up readily under one's fingers. Tumors on the anterior wall may be indistinguishable from the symphysis and tumors on the posterior wall in women may frequently be mistaken for the uterus."

The bimanual examination is an important aspect in clinical staging and should be performed with the full realization that findings may significantly influence therapy. The lesion may not be palpable or there may be an apparent asymmetrical spongy feel to the bladder. This latter finding is frequent with multiple, non-infiltrating tumors. Because the tumor is palpable does not automatically mean that it is infiltrating. With infiltration, there is usually a sensation of induration or bladder wall thickening as well. The mass moves with the bladder and does not seem to slip about inside the bladder. Perivesical tumors feel larger than they appear on cystoscopic examinations; they are nodular or project from the surface of the bladder wall and are mobile in the pelvis. The characteristic difference between muscular and perivesical tumors lies in the hard, nodular surface of the latter.[273] Fixation of the tumor in the pelvis indicates Stage D disease.

*twenty-two*

---

# Chapter 4

# Natural History, Staging and Grading, and Pathology

**B**LADDER tumors constitute a heterogeneous problem, a complex group of conditions with different etiologies, a long spectrum of clinical courses, and variable responses to treatment; Friedman,[107] for example, has listed 12 distinct clinicopathological types. The natural history of a solitary papillary tumor arising from the lateral or posterior wall differs from a similar one located at the bladder neck or urethral orifice. Tumors in the lateral locations invade easily and spread more rapidly; they usually cause symptoms relatively early, however. The bladder dome is readily accessible to operative procedures (TUR or partial cystectomy), but tumors located at that site usually remain silent until of considerable size; as a consequence, when discovered, they already may be non-resectable. The cells of a sessile tumor have a broader base for invasion than do similar cells in a tumor with a narrow stalk. Solid tumors infiltrate readily; such tumors in the trigone have a particularly ominous outlook. An infected, ulcerated neoplasm presents additional difficulties during treatment and subsequent healing, which may be prolonged.

Staging and histologic grading of bladder tumors are impor-

*twenty-three*

tant to assist in deciding the treatment most suitable and in predicting prognosis. The accuracy of clinical staging depends on the thoroughness of investigations utilized. Clinical staging is based primarily on cystoscopic observations, bimanual examination, and radiologic investigations. Histologic findings are of importance as well; in fact, often this is a major criterion used for staging since it is less subjective than the other commonly used clinical methods. Nevertheless, staging that is based primarily on the degree of infiltration demonstrated on transurethral biopsy specimens is subject to significant error, since often it is not possible to biopsy adequately the depth of the lesion and hence the real extent of infiltration is not determined. And depth of infiltration is the most important factor effecting treatment and prognosis.

The three most common methods currently in vogue for staging carcinoma of the bladder are the staging recognized by the British Institute of Urology (Pugh),[228] the Marshall modification of the Jewett and Strong classification,[144, 184, 185] and that of the Unio Internationalis Contra Cancrum (U.I.C.C.).[181, 244] With the former classification, mucosal tumors are Stage $T_1$, muscular tumors are Stage $T_2$, perivesical tumors are Stage $T_3$, and Stage $T_4$ lesions show pelvic fixation or distant metastases. There is no distinction made between superficial or deep muscle involvement. In the Marshall classification, a Stage O lesion is limited to the mucosa. A Stage A lesion does not extend beyond the submucosa. Superficial muscle invasion is noted in Stage $B_1$ tumors and deep muscle involvement is apparent in Stage $B_2$ lesions. Stage C neoplasms extend into the perivesical tissues. Spread to the pelvis is noted in Stage $D_1$ lesions; there is spread outside the pelvis in Stage $D_2$ lesions.

The U.I.C.C. staging system is outlined in Table 4-I where it is compared with the other classifications. Therapy and prognosis are perhaps best guided by this scheme. Since it is a clinical staging classification (with the exception of histologic proof of malignancy), no mention is made of lymph node involvement. This is considered, however, in the U.I.C.C. pathological staging classification, which, incidently, otherwise is identical to the clinical staging system. Whitmore[293] has considered tumors

TABLE 4-I

## COMMONLY USED STAGING CLASSIFICATIONS

| | Papilloma | Mucosal (In Situ) | Infiltrating Submucosal | Infiltrating Superficial Musculature | Involving Deep Musculature | Perivesical Involvement | Fixed to Pelvis or Invading Adjacent Organs | Distant Metastases |
|---|---|---|---|---|---|---|---|---|
| British Institute of Urology (Pugh)[228] | | $T_1$ | $T_1$ | $T_2$ | $T_2$ | $T_3$ | $T_4$ | $T_4$ |
| Marshall Modification of Jewett and Strong Classification[184] | | O | A | $B_1$ | $B_2$ | C | $D_1$* | $D_2$ |
| U.I.C.C.[181, 244] | $T_x$ | $T_{is}$ | $T_1$ | $T_2$ | $T_3$ | $T_3$ | $T_4$ | $T_4$ |
| Whitmore[293] | (..Superficial............) | | | (..Deep............) | | | (..Metastatic.....) | |

* Pelvic fixation not included in Marshall classification; Lymph node involvement considered instead, but this ordinarily can be ascertained only at operation.

as either superficial, deep, or metastatic as indicated in Table 4-I. Prognosis is readily predictable with this simple classification; survival diminishes markedly with deep muscle involvement or perivesical extension and further decreases with metastatic disease.

Most consider prostatic involvement a justification for a Stage $T_4$ or $D_1$ classification. Urologists are inclined to this course since prostatic involvement adversely effects the results of cystectomy, the patients with spread to the prostate behaving as patients with Stage $T_4$ or $D_1$ tumors; e.g., Marshall had no survivors among 20 patients with prostatic involvement even though 9 of these had negative pelvic lymph nodes. Patients with extension of tumor to the prostate treated by irradiation tend to behave more like patients with clinical Stage $T_3$ or C tumors and therefore will be so classified by myself. In the Stanford series,[48] 3 of 16 patients with prostatic involvement were alive and well at 3 years.

In 1952, Marshall[184] presented his modification of the Jewett and Strong classification for staging bladder tumors. At the same

TABLE 4-II

RELATIONSHIP OF CLINICAL AND SURGICAL STAGING (MARSHALL)[184]

*Clinical Stage = A and B$_1$ (29 cases)*
1)  5 were pathologically Stage O
2) 14 were pathologically Stage A or B$_1$
3)  7 were pathologically Stage B$_2$ or C
4)  3 were pathologically Stage D

*Clinical Stage = B$_2$ and C (67 cases)*
1)  0 were pathologically Stage O
2)  9 were pathologically Stage A or B$_1$
3) 25 were pathologically Stage B$_2$ or C
4) 33 were pathologically Stage D

*Clinical Stage = D (8 cases)*
1)  0 were pathologically Stage O
2)  1 were pathologically Stage A or B$_1$
3)  2 were pathologically Stage B$_2$ or C
4)  5 were pathologically Stage D

*NOTE:* Low grade lesions were usually not over-estimated if they were clinical Stage A or B$_1$ and high grade lesions usually were not overestimated if they were clinical Stage B$_2$ or C.

time, he compared the relationship of clinical staging to surgical staging based on 104 consecutive patients having radical cystectomy, all clinically staged prior to cystectomy. Table 4-II shows the results of this comparison. In 42 per cent of the cases, the pathologic stage was greater than the clinical appraisal (clinically underestimated). In 16 per cent, the cases were pathologically staged lower than the clinical staging (clinically overestimated). The discrepancy was greatest for the clinical Stage B$_2$ and C lesion: 33 of 67 cases so staged were pathologically Stage D. *This discrepancy between the clinical stage and surgical stage is important when evaluating treatment results, for patients with operatively or pathologically staged lesions will have a better prognosis, stage for stage, than patients with clinically staged tumors.* Recent experience indicates that clinical staging is now somewhat more reliable for transitional cell carcinomas with approximately 75 per cent of all tumors being correctly staged.[273] The presence of clinically unrecognizable pelvic lymph nodes is the most frequent reason for understaging. Inflammation is the major cause for overstaging. Because of the proclivity for spread outside the bladder, squamous cell carcinomas and other less frequently seen tumors, such as sarcomas, are understaged 40 to 45 per cent of the time.

In spite of the shortcomings of clinical staging, it has proved of value in guiding therapy and in predicting prognosis. Clinical staging is based on information which can be obtained in all cases during the course of a clinical evaluation. Subsequent information obtained by operative intervention or post mortem examination cannot alter the clinical stage. More satisfactory comparison of results in different series of cases treated by different methods is possible if, as a minimum, clinical staging is used. Reporting cases by operative stage alone makes comparison with radiotherapy cases impossible.

Three hundred and three cases of infiltrating carcinoma of the bladder were critically studied by Jewett and Eversole;[143] 252 cases were suitable for analysis. Sections had been taken from specimens obtained at cystectomy, segmental resection, and autopsy. Lymphatics were found to be invaded at some level of the bladder wall in 87 cases. They were involved in only

7 of 62 instances in which the tumor had failed to extend to the halfway level in the muscle wall: of these 7, only 2, both poorly differentiated squamous cancers, metastasized to a depth greater than that reached by the primary growth. Local lymphatic involvement for different stages was as follows: Stage A, 1 in 40; Stage $B_1$, 6 in 22; Stage $B_2$, 14 in 35; Stage C, 66 in 155.

The tumors were found to penetrate the wall of the bladder in three characteristic ways. The tendency was for most of them to invade as a more or less compact mass in any direction from the main tumor (70 per cent of 252 cases). The chief exception was in the cases of poorly differentiated squamous carcinoma that were deeply invasive. In these, the characteristic pattern consisted of fingerlike projections of invasive tumor, often cut across in such a way as to appear in sections as isolated clumps or nests, which in all but a very few cases lay within one or two low power microscopic fields of the main tumor (27 per cent of 252 cases). Isolated, individual infiltrating cells were seen rarely. Cells also invaded as intramural lymphatic metastases, traveling in a direction more or less perpendicular to the plane of the overlying bladder mucosa (3 per cent). Mostofi[207] found similar patterns of spread although he found lymphatic invasion more frequently than did Jewett and Eversole.[143] Errors in the preoperative estimate of extent of infiltration usually were found among cases exhibiting either the fingerlike projections of invasion or the intramural lymphatic metastases.

Simon, Cordonnier, and Snodgrass[251] found lymphatic channel invasion in 9 of 38 bladders studied with sections of 11 portions of each bladder removed at cystectomy. Lymphatic involvement usually was in close proximity to the principal tumor mass. Three of these nine patients were still alive at the time of the report; two had no evidence of recurrence after $1\frac{1}{2}$ years, but the third had evidence of recurrence. All of the nine were very malignant, invasive carcinomas, penetrating deeply into the muscle and in most cases, into fat. No lymphatic invasion was seen with superficial tumors (12 Stage A and 7 Stage $B_1$). Three bladders were found to contain previously unnoticed and grossly undetectable carcinoma *in situ* far removed from the principal tumor mass. Transurethral resection or partial cystectomy would not have removed these minute carcinomas.

Baker[6] evaluated carefully the spread of bladder tumors in cystectomy specimens. If tumors were extending less than halfway through the bladder wall, one of five patients had positive lymph nodes in the pelvis. In two instances, tumor was noted in the bladder wall lymphatics up to a distance of six times the diameter of the primary tumor. Ten cystectomy specimens also were available in which there was tumor extension more than halfway through the bladder wall. Eight of these had positive pelvic lymph nodes. Circumferential spread of tumor in lymphatics involving up to 60 per cent of the bladder was noted. Spread from these lymphatics to vesicular and regional lymphatics usually follows promptly.

Jewett and Strong[144] summated data from autopsies on 127 cases of infiltrating tumors of the bladder. In a group of 15 patients with Stage B tumors, bladder wall lymphatic invasion was noted in only one patient and in another regional metastases were present. There were 89 cases with perivesical involvement, Stage C patients; vesical wall lymphatics only were involved in six instances. Regional or distant metastases were noted in 52; 19 had distant metastases without apparent regional lymph node metastases.

The regional lymph nodes were involved in 64 per cent of the cases, the liver in 50 per cent, the lungs in 34 per cent, and the bones in 21 per cent. Skin metastases were occasionally seen. Melicow[196] and Maltry[182] reported similar findings. Wallace[273] indicates poorly differentiated papillary lesions show a great affinity for hepatic spread while well differentiated papillary carcinomata metastasize more frequently to bone and lung.

Lymphatic spread of tumor from the dome is to external iliac, hypogastric and common iliac lymph nodes. The trigonal and lateral wall tumors, perhaps representing 70 per cent of all bladder neoplasms, spread to the obturator and external iliac lymph nodes primarily. Anterior tumors also spread to the external iliac lymph nodes while posterior cancers spread to the external iliac as well as retrofemoral, hypogastric and presacral lymph nodes.

*twenty-nine*

In males, invasion of the prostate is common since about 50 per cent of tumors involve the trigone. A slightly higher incidence of bone metastases has been reported when the prostate and seminal vesicles were invaded by a bladder tumor. Bone metastases actually may be more frequent than figures indicate since thorough examination of the skeletal system is not always carried out. Melicow[196] concluded from his review that in a patient with a tumor whose primary origin was in doubt, i.e., bladder or prostate, the mere presence of radiographic evidence of bone involvement did not necessarily favor the prostate as the primary site.

Friedell and McAuley[105] recently reported on 31 patients with untreated bladder carcinoma. All cases were autopsied. Two-thirds of the patients whose ages ranged from 47 to 89 years, developed urinary symptoms less than a year before death; one had had urinary symptoms, perhaps the result of bladder cancer, for 9 years. Metastases were found in 20 cases with the regional lymph nodes (16), lung (7), liver (5), and bone (5) most frequently involved. Metastases were seen in 4 of 10 cases with Stage $B_1$ bladder disease, 7 of 9 cases with Stage $B_2$, and 9 of 12 with Stage C. All but 1 of 21 patients with Stage $B_2$ or C bladder disease had metastases or blood vessel invasion. Pelvic organs, particularly the prostate (11) and seminal vesicles (8), were involved by direct extension in 20 cases. Renal insufficiency, sepsis and pneumonia were the most common causes of death. These findings parallel those of Sauer and associates[241] in 60 cases of untreated bladder cancer.

Yet even with the propensity of bladder tumors for distant spread, Caldwell, Bagshaw, and Kaplan[48] and others[118, 198, 235] have found persistent disease in the bladder or pelvis a frequent cause for treatment failure. This group of patients is potentially curable. Improvement in local treatment may salvage a greater percentage than at present.

In Kurohara's[156, 157] review of bladder cancer he found that approximately 70 per cent of patients dying of bladder cancer have residual tumor as the cause of death. Complications of treatment account for 10 to 15 per cent of deaths (1 per cent for irradiation to as high as 21 per cent for cystectomy), and

*thirty*

TABLE 4-III

| | |
|---|---|
| *Papilloma* | Small, single papillary tumor with a slender main pedicle.<br>Normal polarity of cells on well defined and intact basement membrane without infiltration.<br>Mitotic figures absent or very scarce. |
| *Grade I* | Gross character of a papilloma.<br>Slight loss of polarity of cells and atypical appearance or arrangement of cells.<br>Basement membrane intact.<br>Few mitoses. |
| *Grade II* | Multiple papillary tumors with slender pedicles or a large papillary tumor with a thick pedicle.<br>Loss of polarity and atypical appearance (in 25-50 per cent) and arrangement of cells.<br>Areas of basement membrane may be lost, but obvious infiltration of the pedicle or bladder wall is not demonstrable. |
| *Grade III* | Obviously infiltrating papillary tumor or carcinoma in which the papillary structure is recognizable, but most of the cells are atypical in appearance (50-75 per cent) and arrangement. |
| *Grade IV* | Non-papillary, infiltrating tumor.<br>Practically all cells atypical in appearance. |

15 to 20 per cent die of other diseases (31 per cent for irradiation and 2 per cent for cystectomy). Of those patients dying, local persistence of cancer was found in various series to be the cause of death in from 9 to 60 per cent of the cases. Widespread disease was found the cause in from 15 to 53 per cent of cases. Baker[8] reported that 32 per cent of patients with Stage A lesions, 33 per cent of those with Stage $B_1$ disease, and 85 per cent of the cases with Stage $B_2$ or C cancer, die with cancer.

Grading of tumor has two major classifications. The Broders'[38, 230] classification (Table 4-III) is used most frequently in this country. Grading is based on the surgeon's description of the tumor and the histologic findings. A papilloma is a mucosal tumor with typical characteristics as shown in Figure 4-1. Grade I and II tumors (Figs. 4-2A and 2B) are of low grade, whereas Grade III and IV tumors (Figs. 4-3A and 3B) are poorly differentiated and are considered high grade tumors. Beautiful color histological photographs of bladder tumors appear in the

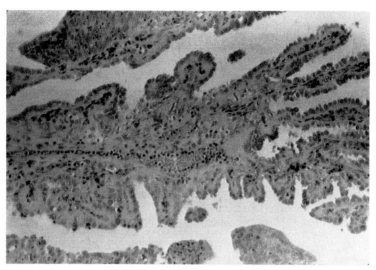

FIGURE 4-1. Papilloma: Transitional cell epithelium is normal in appearance. A delicate connective tissue stroma is present. (×160)

Armed Forces' Institute of Pathology monograph by Friedman and Ash.[110] The low grade tumors are ordinarily low stage tumors as well and the high grade lesions are usually infiltrative and therefore in higher stages (Fig. 4-4).

Pugh's[228] histologic grading system (Table 4-IV) also is useful; it has been adopted by the British Institute of Urology. Papillomas are considered benign tumors; "the papilloma is covered by a layer of transitional epithelium that is indistinguishable from the normal bladder mucosa, whereas in the differentiated transitional cell carcinoma, the cells are usually larger and plumper and often vary in size and may be irregularly hyperchromatic. Mitoses occur quite frequently." Transitional cell carcinoma is classified as either differentiated or anaplastic. Squamous cell carcinoma and adenocarcinoma are rare; they account for only 2 per cent of the tumors in Pugh's series of over 1,400 cases. Glandular or squamous metaplasia often is seen, occurring with greater frequency in anaplastic than in differentiated tumors. Multiple primary tumors with different histopathology are seen occasionally.[121, 254]

Four pathologic characteristics are considered important by

*thirty-two*

Jewett.[141] These are depth of infiltration, histological pattern, grade of malignancy, and invasion of the lymphatics or veins within the wall of the bladder. These features establish the essential nature of the neoplasm and help to predict prognosis as well as guide therapy. McDonald and Thompson[176] place much emphasis on vascular invasion, either perineural lymphatic involvement or venous invasion, since the presence of same adversely influences prognosis.

Before deciding upon the specific therapeutic approach in a

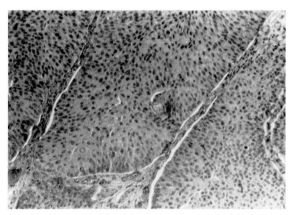

FIGURE 4-2A. Grade I transitional cell carcinoma: Well ordered pattern of cells; few mitoses evident. (×160)

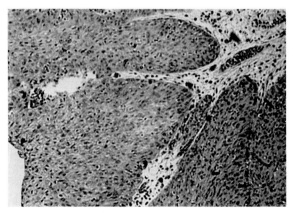

FIGURE 4-2B. Grade II transitional cell carcinoma. Loss of polarity seen. Cellular atypism is prominent. (×160)

*thirty-three*

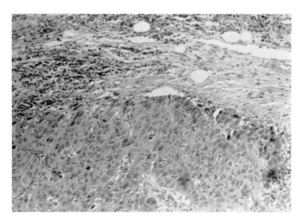

FIGURE 4-3A. Grade III transitional cell carcinoma. Frequent mitoses, cellular atypism and loss of polarity are all important features (×160)

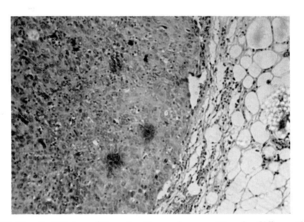

FIGURE 4-3B. Grade IV transitional cell carcinoma. Poorly differentiated cells are seen which invade paravesical fat. Mitotic activity is very evident.

specific patient, the urologist or radiotherapist needs specific information about what Mostofi[207] calls the "degree of malignancy." The degree of malignancy is assessed by the histologic characteristics of the tumor, degree of anaplasia, growth pattern, depth of infiltration and mode and location of local spread.

Histologically, 90 per cent of tumors are transitional cell carcinomas, 6 to 7 per cent are true squamous cell carcinomas, and 1 to 2 per cent are adenocarcinomas. Other cell types are rare.

*thirty-four*

Foci of squamous cell carcinoma or, less frequently, adeno-carcinoma may be seen in transitional cell carcinoma. Such histologic findings should be reported since they have prognostic as well as possible epidemiological significance.

Grading is ordinarily based on the degree of anaplasia. Variations in size, shape, and staining characteristics of cells, frequency and type of mitotic figures, and presence of abnormal cells all categorize the degree of anaplasia. High grade neoplasms show marked anaplasia and low grade lesions have minimal anaplastic change. Although high grade lesions are often infiltrative, the depth of infiltration does not directly relate to the degree of anaplasia.

Tumors should be described as being papillary, infiltrating, papillary and infiltrating, or nonpapillary and noninfiltrating. These features have an important bearing on treatment as well as prognosis.

Depth of infiltration effects prognosis more than any other single feature of bladder cancer. The level of deepest infiltra-

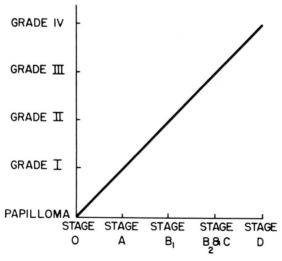

FIGURE 4-4. The relationship of histological grade and state of disease. Rarely is there more than one category of deviation from the indicated line.

| | |
|---|---|
| Papilloma | |
| Differentiated | |
| Anaplastic | Transitional cell carcinoma |
| Squamous cell carcinoma | |
| Adenocarcinoma | |
| Other varieties of malignant tumors | |

tion demonstrated on pathological evaluation should be reported.

As stated earlier in this chapter, local spread occurs either by *en bloc* invasion, tentacular invasion, or by lymphatic invasion. Mostofi noted lymphatic channel involvement in 40 per cent of deeply infiltrating tumors; such invasion is usually readily recognized. Lymphatic spread is more difficult to detect in superficial and low grade lesions.

Fahmy[93] has reported recently on histologic features of urinary bladder tumors based on a study of 411 urinary bladder biopsies. Only 4 per cent of the biopsies showed benign papillomas, 56 per cent of the cases showed differentiated transitional cell carcinoma and 28 per cent of the cases showed anaplastic transitional cell carcinoma. Squamous cell carcinoma was found in approximately 4 per cent of the patients and adenocarcinoma represented less than 1 per cent.

The frequency of the squamous cell tumors depends on one's criteria for establishing such a diagnosis. Fahmy[93] insists that a squamous cell carcinoma be diagnosed only if there is no papillary transitional cell component. Squamous cell metaplasia, even pronounced, in a papillary tumor is not considered enough to grade it as a squamous cell carcinoma. Mostofi[206] classified 10 per cent of the bladder tumors in his series as being squamous cell carcinomas and an additional 15 to 20 per cent of transitional cell carcinomas showed areas with squamous epithelium.

Eighty-four cases of squamous cell carcinoma of the bladder were reviewed by Newman and associates.[210] One-fourth of the tumors were squamous cell carcinomas mixed with transitional or adenocarcinoma patterns; some pathologists might have classified these as other than squamous cell carcinomas. Based on Broders' tumor grading, 88 per cent of the cancers were grade 3 or 4; 46 per cent showed lymphatic or vascular invasion in the pathologic specimen at the time of the initial examination.

The adenocarcinomas of the bladder which arise in the anterior wall and dome are urachal in origin; they are principally intramural with frequent extravesical extensions.[14] Adenocarcinomas occurring elsewhere in the bladder may be more difficult to diagnose since the tumor may contain mostly mucin with either little or no epithelium or well-differentiated cells. Deep biopsy may be necessary to confirm the diagnosis.[207]

Bladder tumors in children are predominantly mesothelial in origin. Sarcoma botryoides, a polypoid rhabdomyosarcoma histologically, is diagnosed most frequently.[250] Myosarcomas of the bladder are very rare; MacKenzie and associates[175] reported on the Memorial Hospital experiences with this tumor type in 20 cases seen from 1920 to 1967. Seven of these were in patients 10 years of age or less.

Melicow[196] analyzed the clinical and pathologic features of over 2,500 specimens and biopsies of tumors of the urinary bladder. This excellent review should be read in its entirety by those seriously concerned with the bladder tumor problem. He feels that the pathologic diagnosis is preferably given in the form of a complete sentence; for example, "well differentiated, non-infiltrating, papillary carcinoma of the urinary bladder, Grade I" or "poorly differentiated, infiltrating carcinoma of the urinary bladder with invasion of the superficial muscularis, Grade II." The majority of his patients of bladder tumors were found to be papillary (81 per cent of the cases); 12 per cent of the papillary tumors were considered papillomas which means that 10 per cent of all of the bladder tumors were considered papillomas.

In the Institute of Urology series reported by Pugh,[228] only 3 per cent of the patients had benign papillomas and Mostofi[206] classified 3 per cent of his tumors as being benign papillomas. Fahmy[93] considered 4 per cent of the bladder tumors in his series as papillomas. These series of cases show considerably fewer benign papillomas than most reports; as noted earlier, their criteria of benignancy are quite rigid. A papilloma is considered a pathological classification and such a diagnosis is not justified for a benign looking, papillary, pedunculated tumor seen at cystoscopy, without biopsy confirmation.[5]

The histological diagnosis of cancer is ordinarily made on the basis of cellular anaplasia, invasion and metastasis. Since most bladder tumors metastasize relatively late and superficial invasion is difficult to detect early because a well defined basement membrane is not seen in bladder mucosa, anaplasia is the feature which must be relied upon for establishing a diagnosis of superficial bladder cancer. Criteria of anaplasia established by the American Bladder Tumor Registry and the World Health Organization include: increased cellularity, nuclear crowding, disturbances of cellular polarity, failure of differentiation from base to surface, polymorphism, irregularity in the size of cells, variation in the shape of nuclei and their chromatin pattern, presence of giant cells, and displaced or abnormal mitotic figures. Such changes may occasionally be seen in regenerative or reactive conditions of the bladder mucosa.[207]

Without using rigid restrictive criteria for establishing a diagnosis of papilloma, many papillary tumors will be called benign when in actual fact they are malignant. Nichols and Marshall[212] found that carcinoma developed in 7 of their 42 patients with a diagnosis of benign papilloma histologically.

Histological material on 82 cases of bladder papillomas (contributor's diagnosis) submitted to the U. S. Armed Forces Institute of Pathology were reviewed. Only 24 of these cases were considered by Dean[71] to be papillomas. He found that even with stringent rules applied for diagnosing papilloma (either invasion or anaplasia) that 5 of these 24 patients diagnosed as having benign papilloma were dead of cancer within 5 years. The excluded cases did less well. As a result of findings of this sort, many pathologists are reluctant to even consider diagnosing benign papilloma since their behavior is so unpredictable. Nevertheless, others have apparently had a reasonable success in selecting out benign tumors. Bergkvist,[15] for example, found that only one of the 64 patients thought to have benign papillomas died within 5 years with cancer; 21 per cent of the bladder tumors in his series of 300 cases, incidentally, were considered benign papillomas. In the series of bladder tumors reported by Chapman and Sutherland,[50] 37.5 per cent were diagnosed as simple papillomas (Grade O) and at the Urological Clinic of the Salford Royal Hospital in Manchester, England, 58 per cent of patients with vesical tumors were classified as having benign papillomata.[221] These reports contrast sharply with the 3 per cent incidence of papillomata reported by Mostofi[206] and Pugh[228] and the 4 per cent by Fahmy;[93] 10 per cent of bladder tumors evaluated by Melicow[196] were considered papillomas.

Considerable evidence is presented by Melicow[196] to substantiate his view that many of the so-called "recurrences" of bladder tumors following fulguration are really new tumor formations. Of 205 bladder tumors which were initially single, approximately 70 per cent returned with tumors; almost half of these were multiple. In many instances, "recurrences" were in areas other than that of the primary tumor. The carcinogenic factors responsible for the initial tumor presumably continue to be active even after successful treatment of a single lesion.

Neoplasia of the urothelium may involve any part of the urinary tract that is exposed to urine. These changes may be secondary to seeding of cells in the urine, but certainly in many cases continued exposure to carcinogens must be an etiologic factor. Schade and Swinney[243] found precancerous abnormalities in the mucosa away from the primary tumor in 80 of 100 cases of transitional cell carcinoma; carcinoma *in situ* was noted in 40 instances. Lymphatic spread of tumors also may play a role. The true nature of this process needs further explanation.

In reviewing his material, Wallace[278] found a high incidence of multiple lesions when there was a long survival period for follow-up. In all patients followed after nephro-ureterectomy for renal cell carcinoma, lesions developed in the bladder, some after an interval of 14 years before being recognized in the bladder. In his cystectomy series, where the ureters were examined routinely, there was a 10 per cent incidence of either *in situ* or invasive tumors within the last four inches of the ureter. Gowing[119] reported on post-mortem findings of patients who at one time had had a bladder neoplasm. When the urethra was fixed immediately after death, 20 per cent showed demonstrable lesions of carcinoma *in situ* at that site; these lesions apparently did not represent implants, but instead were interpreted as being independent neoplastic foci. He found 5 per cent of the bladder tumors also with tumors in one renal pelvis or ureter; often both ureters were involved.

Carcinoma *in situ* of the bladder is a well defined entity.[2, 120, 194] The epithelium in this condition is composed of cells that look like cancer cells, but there is no invasion of the poorly defined basement membrane. Melamed[193] in this country reported on 25 patients with carcinoma *in situ* of the bladder. The disease progressed to invasive cancer in 9 of the 25 patients during the course of the study. The time required for development was a median of 26 months, with a maximum of 67 months. Table 4-V shows the schematic diagram which Melamed[192] uses to describe the pathogenesis of this process.

Melamed[193] has defined clearly the pathologic criteria for the diagnosis of *in situ* carcinoma which is essentially similar to that for *in situ* carcinoma of organs with squamous epithelium. "The most striking and consistent feature is disproportionate nuclear enlargement and hyperchromasia in epithelial cells. This may be variable from cell to cell giving an overall disorderly appearance, or it may be almost uniform throughout the epithelium. Individual nuclei are often irregular or angular in configuration rather than smoothly round or ovoid. Mitoses are present, but not necessarily numerous or abnormal. There may be some variation in overall cell size with cytoplasmic

TABLE 4-V

PATHOGENESIS OF BLADDER CARCINOMA (MELAMED)[192]

Carcinogen Exposure
↓
Cytologically Normal Phase (Clinically Normal)
↓
Cytologically Abnormal Phase (Clinically Normal)
↓
Clinical Carcinoma

*forty*

vacuolization or increased eosinophilia, but cytoplasmic changes are otherwise not remarkable. Because of diminished intercellular cohesion, the epithelium sometimes takes on a loose appearance."

Patients with *in situ* disease can be detected by cytologic screening of their urine. Cytologic screening has proven very helpful in following high risk patients.[276] In the rubber industry in Great Britain, routine cytologic screening has resulted in 63 asymptomatic tumors being detected in 80,000 examinations of urine. Furthermore, there have been apparently positive smears when no tumor was recognizable cystoscopically and many other non-malignant lesions have been detected as a result of this screening. Careful screening is essential; expert cytology is as important as expert cystoscopy. The average incidence of false positives is approximately 2 to 3 per cent; these usually occur in patients with severe chronic cystitis or in patients with urinary calculi. The method is best suited for poorly differentiated tumors and is more accurate for recurrent carcinomas than for primary tumors.[152] Cytologic evaluation may be particularly helpful in patients with diverticula which cannot be visualized cystoscopically. Also, it is helpful in diagnosing non-papillary carcinomas which may be mistaken cystoscopically for cystitis.[264]

Ultraviolet tetracycline fluorescence has been used in an effort to detect *in situ* carcinoma.[195, 292] Tetracycline is incorporated into metabolically active tissues and such tissues containing tetracycline will fluoresce when exposed to ultraviolet light. Tetracycline (250 mg.) is ordinarily given every four hours for at least two days. The drug is then discontinued for 24 to 36 hours before examination. *In situ* lesions, as well as invasive cancer, have been found by this technique in bladder mucosa that appears either normal or only inflamed by ordinary light cystoscopy. In 7 patients, Whitmore and Bush[289] found a total of 12 areas of bladder cancer identified by tetracycline ultraviolet fluorescence in areas where the bladder mucosa appeared either normal or had only an inflamed appearance by visible light cystoscopy. Eighteen of 21 proven cancers demonstrated fluorescence, whereas only 2 of 13 papillomas fluoresced. Melamed[194] has noted that in areas with histologically proven carcinoma *in situ* there may not necessarily be fluorescence either. Tetracycline fluorescence also may give additional information as to the true extent of the tumor.

Histological techniques, such as those introduced by Veenema and associates,[268] may develop to the degree that therapy will be influenced thereby. *In vitro* autoradiography can select with reasonable certainty the tumors which have either poor or good prognosis, poor prognosis being seen in patients with tumors with high activity. There is rough correlation between the tritiated thymidine autoradiograph activity and histological grade.

Lamb[159] has noted that tumors with a normal chromosome count did not ordinarily infiltrate. When there was a spread of the chromosome count or when the count was in the 92 to 96 range, infiltration was almost always demonstrable. His study described the chromosome counts and the histologic features of 30 transitional cell carcinomas of the bladder. With progressive loss of cellular differentiation, there is first: 1) an increase and then a decrease in the chromosome number; 2) a wider range of chromosome numbers, and 3) an increase in chromosome structural abnormalities. The appearance of invasion is related more closely to an increase in the chromosome count than the loss of cellular differentiation. Wallace[277] raises the question as to whether radiotherapy may change the chromosome count of tumors. On reviewing histories of patients with multiple papillomatosis of the bladder treated by radioactive sodium or bromine, most of whom were of a well differentiated grade, 40 per cent died subsequently of distant metastases. This cytogenetic approach ultimately may be refined sufficiently to assist selection of therapy utilized.

*Chapter 5*

---

# Philosophy of Treatment

PATIENTS with untreated tumors of the bladder have a
bad prognosis; less than 4 per cent in Prout and Marshall's[226] series of 59 such cases collected over a 20-year period
lived more than 5 years after diagnosis. Sauer and associates[142]
reported in 1950 on 60 cases of untreated bladder cancer; 90
per cent were dead within a year and there were no 2 year survivors. More recently, Friedell and McAuley[105] reported on 31
untreated autopsy cases with similar findings. Clearly, this is a
virulent tumor; some sort of treatment is usually indicated.

As in the treatment of any disease, guidance for therapy is
obtained from one's own past experience as well as that of others as reported in the literature. Unfortunately, it is still ex-
tremely difficult to evaluate treatment results and determine
from them the therapy of choice in other cases. This is because
of the absence of uniformity in the classification of malignant
lesions in terms of pathology, degree of malignancy, extent, and
location, all of which require consideration in determining the
most suitable treatment and in ascertaining results. Differences
in staging (e.g., clinical staging versus operative or pathologic
staging) and in selection factors between various reported se-

ries makes meaningful comparison of treatment methods impossible.

Current opinions regarding the treatment of carcinoma of the bladder are widely divergent and for the most part are based on personal opinion rather than on well established data. As Otis noted in 1888, "no author has a right to claim a settlement of important practical points on his own bare assertion; to contradict the results of a large and carefully tabulated experience by the citation of one or two cases."[185] Yet, such license is still frequently taken in the literature and in clinical practice. Unfortunately, at present no good controlled series are available to definitely assist in establishing treatment guidelines for the varied types of bladder tumors.

Any rational treatment policy must be based on knowledge of the natural history of the particular tumor being evaluated. The location and size of the tumor, its histology, the tumor stage, and the general condition of the patient are all important considerations. As Melicow[196] has indicated, "it is not possible in the present state of our knowledge to be dogmatic as to the superiority of one form of therapy over the other, but it is important to know the nature of the enemy, to understand the problem, and the indications, effectiveness, and limitations of all the modalities of therapy; that is half the battle."

Jewett[140] has assessed the problem as follows: "The causes of disagreement concerning the efficacy of the therapeutic procedures in current use for treatment of carcinoma of the bladder have their origin primarily in one's failure to duplicate, with a certain method of treatment, the good results reported by others, or to obtain good results consistently. This failure nearly always is attributable to one or more of three variables. These are: 1) the limitations inherent in the procedure that was used; 2) a lack of expertness in the technical application of the procedure, and 3) the differences in curability of the tumors concerned. These causes of therapeutic failure are subject to such wide variation that the value of each, in any given situation, is difficult to assess. Different procedures may not be equally applicable to all potentially curable tumors."

Wallace[278] believes "bladder tumors can be handled in a positive or a negative fashion, managed or mismanaged. Among the causes of mismanagement are the following: a) Inadequate appreciation of the gravity of the situation when a tumor is diagnosed as a papilloma without histologic confirmation and when procrastination is permitted before treatment in the belief that the tumor is in fact benign. The genuine papilloma that runs a benign course is a relatively rare tumor. All bladder tumors should be considered to be malignant until proved otherwise. b) Inadequate assessment so that conservative surgery is attempted when a tumor on more complete examination would be recognized as being beyond the scope of local surgery. Similarly, radical surgery may be mismanagement of a tumor that would have been amenable to more conservative measures. c) Inadequate consultation between urologists and radiotherapists." This last fault in management is particularly obvious in many institutions of this country.

At another time Wallace[280] reiterated these views and hit the heart of several important aspects of the bladder cancer therapy problem. "Early treatment will save patients in whom infiltration is limited, and also cure the lesions where infiltration is not yet apparent—provided they are not made worse by injudicious surgical intervention. Inadequate therapy may convert a tumor with a good biologic potential into one with a bad potential."

The objectives of therapy as well as problems associated with therapy have been discussed succinctly by Melicow.[196] Whenever possible, one should attempt to destroy the cancer with preservation of anatomy and function. When this is not possible one should still attempt to destroy the cancer even if there is moderate sacrifice of anatomy and function associated with such therapy. If such treatment is not possible, then attempts to destroy the cancer even with considerable sacrifice of anatomy and function may be beneficial. In more advanced cases, only palliative therapy is indicated.

Optimal cancer therapy is usually difficult with a limited operative approach to bladder tumors since operation in a contaminated field is ordinarily unavoidable. Furthermore, multiple primaries are frequently present but undetected. Often there are microscopic foci of tumor at a considerable distance from gross tumor at the time of resection, making it difficult to be certain that the margin of resection is adequate. And successful therapy of an established tumor need not mean that carcinogens which are present will not continue to act on the remaining vulnerable urothelium.

Since urologists ordinarily are the first to establish definitely the diagnosis in patients with bladder cancer, they control, in most instances (and certainly so in the United States), the choice of treatment. As a consequence, it is imperative that they remain aware of the established results and potentialities of non-operative management. Particularly in training situations, there is a tendency to lean toward the operative approach, often without real discussion of the possible advantages of non-operative therapy for the patient.

Too frequently, urologists have a lack of appreciation for other treatment modalities. All too often, the attitude toward radiotherapy is as appears in a current *Textbook of Urology*:[187] "external roentgen therapy alone can rarely deliver more than three quarters of an apparently curative dose to the neoplasm without causing so much additional damage as to make this method impractical. Quite properly, new methods of irradiation are being tried and possibly a combination of surgery and irradiation will eventually appear as a method of choice. However, the unwary student can be misled by some of the reports in the literature that are really meant for a more esoteric audience yet do not so indicate. A chronically recurring example is the presentation of a significantly small and heterogeneous group of inadequately defined vesical neoplasms irradiated by means of a theoretically improved machine or technique. Characteristically, the follow-up is merely a current inventory with very few cases of 5 or more years, yet containing a testimonial case and a final aura of hope. Seldom does this case group recognizably appear in the literature 5 years after the patient was treated; and seldom indeed is there a reasonable comparison with similar tumors treated by other means." This opinion is unnecessarily harsh on radiotherapy and is not in keeping with the acts, facts of which all involved in the treatment of bladder must be knowledgeable.

*forty-six*

Sympathetic co-operation between urologists and radiotherapists is essential for the optimal management of patients with carcinoma of the bladder. With the best wishes of the patient always in mind, consideration of all possible forms of therapy is necessary; meaningful, objective interchange between concerned urologists and radiotherapists need be fostered in all situations. Because no one treatment method is acceptable or optimum for all tumors, therapy decisions are difficult in patients with bladder carcinoma. In each patient it is necessary to evaluate the risk of the tumor as compared to the hazards of therapy. Conservative therapy is associated with increased risk of persistence but radical treatment is associated with increased morbidity (often significant morbidity) and mortality.

In the following four chapters, various types of treatment will be presented and evaluated. In the final chapter, treatment recommendations based on these reviews will be suggested.

## Chapter 6

# Radiation Therapy

### A. External Radiotherapy

External ionizing radiations have been used systematically for treating patients with carcinoma of the bladder for more than half a century. In 1905, Gray, in Richmond, Virginia, treated bladder tumors with x-rays administered through a cone inserted through a cystotomy. This method was not used widely, external radiotherapy becoming more commonplace. Numerous five-year cures were recorded in early kilovoltage series; the majority of these, however, were in patients with non-infiltrating tumors. In fact, it was believed for many years that infiltrating carcinoma of the bladder, which was non-resectable, was not curable by irradiation. This proved not an entirely valid assumption since Burnam[41] in 1933 reported 32 five-year cures in 119 patients irradiated for non-resectable bladder cancer. Lower, in the same year, reported 12 five-year cures in 93 non-resectable cases treated with irradiation alone.

Nevertheless, the results of treatment with kilovoltage x-rays were not entirely satisfactory.[95, 218] Clinicians, including radiotherapists, appreciated that this was a virulent tumor requiring

TABLE 6-I

RESULTS OF RADIOTHERAPY (5 YR. SURVIVAL)

| Clinical Stage | St. O, A, B, or $T_1$ Per Cent | St. $B_2$, C or $T_2, T_3$ Per Cent | St. D Per Cent |
|---|---|---|---|
| 1) Dick (64 pts.)[75] | 71 | 9 | 0 |
| 2) Caldwell, Bagshaw, and Kaplan (73 pts.)[48] | 50 | 20 | 0 |
| 3) Jack and Buschke (56 pts.)[137] | 44 | 14 | 0 |
| 4) Ellis (152 pts.)[89] | 36 | 7 | 0 |
| 5) Kurohara, Rubin, and Silon (61 pts.)[157] | 33 | 13 | 0 |
| 6) Crigler, Miller, et al. (126 pts.)[62] | 32 | 28 | 6 |
| 7) Finney and Jones (67 pts.)[98] | 28 | 13 | 0 |
| 8) Van der Werf-Messing (296 pts.)[284] | 12 | 8 | 0 |

aggressive treatment. Farrell and Fetter[94] in 1937 suggested that either more radical surgery be used or larger doses of irradiation be attempted. Normal tissue reactions, particularly those of the skin, produced by kilovoltage x-rays would not permit more aggressive irradiation, however.

Higher irradiation doses did become possible with the availability of megavoltage radiations subsequent to the 1930's; treatment results improved as a consequence. The literature now is replete with series of patients treated either with 1 to 6 mvp x-rays, $^{60}$cobalt gamma rays, or betatron electrons or x-rays with energies of 18 to 35 mev or mvp.[3, 18, 20, 32, 39, 43–45, 48, 60–62, 72, 75, 85, 89, 96, 98, 106, 117, 118, 137, 157, 158, 166, 174, 198, 203, 204, 219, 220, 236, 238, 256, 283, 284, 302]

Table 6-I shows the results or radiotherapy in patients with carcinoma of the bladder, as reported in several of the larger series. The overwhelming majority of these patients were staged clinically. As was discussed in Chapter 4, clinically staged patients will be understaged (when compared with the operative stage) in at least 25 per cent of instances.

The approach to treatment of bladder cancer with irradiation will depend upon the particular situation in a given patient. With Stage A and $B_1$ lesions not suitable for operative treatment or combined resection and radiotherapy, it is probably appropriate to irradiate the bladder only, but with deeply infiltrating tumors (Stage $B_2$ and C) the incidence of lymph node involvement is high and larger fields are required. Particu-

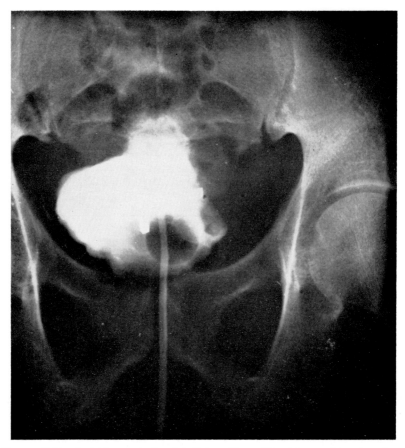

FIGURE 6-1A. Anterior-posterior localizing film with skin markers in place.

larly in females, the posterior urethra may be involved with tumor; it is imperative that this region be irradiated if curative
radiotherapy is initiated.

In every patient treated with external radiations, it is necessary to localize the treatment volume either with fluoroscopy
or with an anterior-posterior film with opaque markers on the
anterior skin (Fig. 6-1A). The bladder is filled with contrast
material (either an iodinated compound such as Hypaque® or
Renovist® or air or carbon dioxide). A horizontal (cross-table)
lateral film also will be required if treatment is to be with other
than an opposed field technique (Fig. 6-1B). In the next para-

graph, dosimetric plots will demonstrate why the opposed field technique is usually an unacceptable treatment method; if 1 to 6 million volt x-rays or [60]cobalt gamma rays are used, the dose to adjacent normal tissue exceeds that of the tumor volume. The volume to be treated is determined from the films and then is drawn onto the patient's cross-sectional contour, obtained in the proposed treatment position. Planning of treatment, to give maximal dose to the required volume and spare apparently uninvolved regions, then is accomplished.[100] The actual computation of plans and the specifics of obtaining the patient's contour are beyond the scope of this monograph, but are clearly described in numerous texts on radiotherapy or radiation physics.

The majority of patients with carcinoma of the bladder treated with megavoltage radiations at this time are irradiated with [60]cobalt gamma rays or with 1 to 6 mvp x-rays. Many patients are irradiated with opposed anterior and posterior fields measuring ordinarily from 10 × 10 cm to perhaps 12 × 12 cm or even 14 × 14 cm in dimensions. The dose distributions from such fields is shown in Figure 6-2A for an average patient with

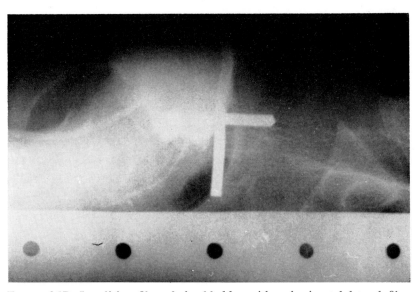

FIGURE 6-1B. Localizing film of the bladder with a horizontal lateral film.

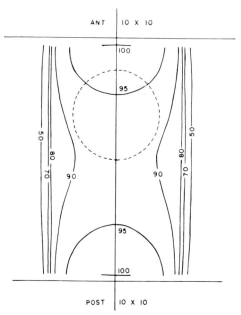

FIGURE 6-2A. Isodose curves for opposed anterior and posterior fields with
⁶⁰cobalt. Dotted line indicates the position of the bladder. Anterior-posterior
diameter 18 cm. The maximum dose (100 per cent) is in the subcutaneous
tissues with only 90 per cent of the maximum to the bladder.

an anterior-posterior diameter of 18 cm and Figure 6-2B shows
the dose distributions with opposed fields for a patient who
measures 26 cm in anterior-posterior dimensions. It is apparent,
particularly for the patient who measures 26 cm, that the dose
distribution is far from ideal. Even though skin sparing is
achieved, there is a higher dose in the subcutaneous and adjacent tissues than in the tumor or bladder. Clearly, such a technique is not acceptable for treating patients in this modern era.
With the three-field technique (Fig. 6-3), using an anterior and
two posterior oblique fields, the maximum dose coincides with
the bladder and tumor. The dose to normal adjacent tissues is
kept below hazardous level.

In certain instances, when it is deemed necessary to treat the
entire pelvis, use of a four-field technique (Fig. 6-4), with opposed anterior and posterior fields as well as opposed lateral
fields, is preferred. The left half of Figure 6-4 demonstrates the

dose distribution in a patient with evenly weighted fields. The right half of Figure 6-4 shows the dose distribution when a third of the radiation is from the anterior field, a third from the posterior field, and a sixth from each of the lateral fields; the dose to the femurs is reduced by this later approach. It is probably necessary to treat patients with clinical Stage $B_2$, C, and D carcinoma of the bladder with such a technique, perhaps adding a supplemental dose to the bladder at the end of treatment using small field rotation therapy.

The dose distribution attained in a typical patient with a

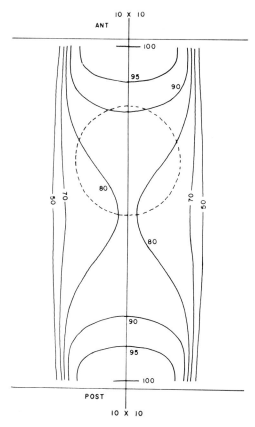

FIGURE 6-2B. As for Figure 6-1A, but anterior-posterior diameter 26 cm. Maximum dose is not in the bladder (tumor volume); in fact, the bladder dose varies from 75 to 90 per cent of the maximum tissue dose.

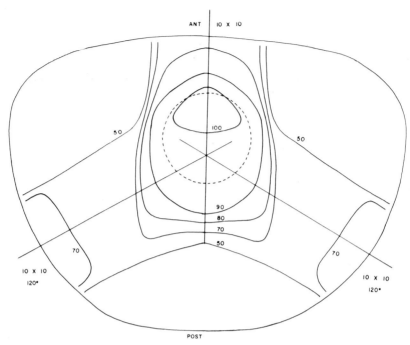

FIGURE 6-3. An improved dose distribution is possible with a 3 field technique, with maximum dose in the bladder. $^{60}$cobalt as in Figure 6-1A and IB.

270° or 360° rotation is shown in Figures 6-5A and 6-5B. In the left half of each contour, the dose distribution is for an 8 × 8 cm field and on the right is for a 12 × 12 cm field. There are certain advantages in the use of the 270° technique, primarily sparing of the rectosigmoid. Also, it is not necessary to treat through the treatment couch with a 270° technique and as a consequence tissue doses are somewhat better defined. As noted, supplemental treatment to the bladder proper can be given by rotation as a central boost to four-field therapy. Patients with Stages A or B$_1$ carcinoma of the bladder can be treated by rotation or with a three-field technique throughout the entire course. Since just the bladder is to be treated, an 8 × 8 cm field is ordinarily sufficiently large. For such patients with superficial bladder tumors treated with small fields it is important that they void before each treatment to reduce the bladder to its minimum volume.

*fifty-four*

Treatment of the bladder is a bit easier with higher energy x-rays, such as those produced by a betatron; a three-field or four-field technique is ordinarily adequate (Fig. 6-6). With such techniques, the maximal irradiation is at the region of concern—the bladder, primary tumor, and, in certain instances, the pelvic lymph nodes.

High energy electrons also have been used in treating patients with bladder carcinoma. Botstein[25] used a single anterior field for a beam with an energy of 35 mev. The dose distribution is such that 80 per cent of the maximal dose is deposited in the posterior bladder (at a depth of 10.5 cm) with approximately 20 per cent of the maximal dose at the mid rectum (a depth of 16 cm). The dose in the anterior abdominal wall, however, by this technique is 100 per cent for a considerable thickness (approximately 6 cm) and patients treated by this method have had considerable subcutaneous reactions secondary to

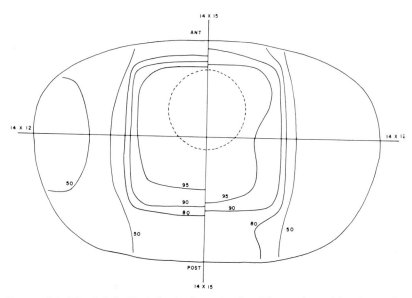

FIGURE 6-4. The left half of the isodose plot is with evenly weighted anterior, posterior and opposed lateral fields with 60cobalt. With a third of the dose from the anterior as well as posterior field, and a sixth from each lateral post, the dose distribution is as shown on the right half. A somewhat improved distribution is evident.

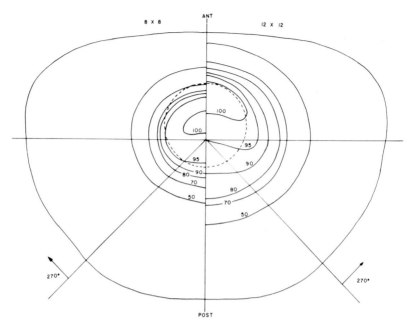

FIGURE 6-5A. 270° rotation with 8 × 8 cm field on the left and 12 × 12 cm field on the right ($^{60}$cobalt). The high dose region flattens from side to side with relative sparing of the posterior structures.

treatment. Figure 6-7 shows an approximate dose distribution from a single anterior electron beam at 35 mev energy.

The dose required to control carcinoma of the bladder is close to the tolerance of normal tissue; with megavoltage radiations, doses equivalent to 6,500 to 7,000 rads in six to seven weeks are necessary. The optimum fractionation and timing of this dose is not as yet precisely determined; it may vary from patient to patient and from tumor to tumor.

Finney[96] showed in patients with clinical Stage $T_1$ and $T_2$ carcinoma (British Institute of Urology classification), a better likelihood of tumor control if treated with daily tumor doses of 300 rads to a total dose of 6,500 rads than with either 200 or 250 rads tumor dose per day, also to a total dose of 6,500 rads. The patients were treated with 4 mvp x-rays using a three-field technique (anterior and two posterior obliques). Table 6-II shows the results of the randomized trial. At three years, 75 per

TABLE 6-II

INFLUENCE OF DAILY DOSE ON TUMOR CONTROL  (FINNEY)[96]

| Daily Tumor Dose (rads) | Number of Cases | Stage | Cases Alive and Well at Two Years | Cases Alive and Well at Three Years |
|---|---|---|---|---|
| 200 | 36 | $T_1$—23% $T_2$—67% | 14/30 | 4/16 |
| 250 | 36 | $T_1$—30% $T_2$—70% | 11/29 | 5/16 |
| 300 | 37 | $T_1$—27% $T_2$—64% $T_3$— 9% | 17/28 | 12/16 |

cent (12/16) of the patients treated with 300 rad increments were alive and well, and only 28 per cent (9/32) survived if treated with tumor doses of 200 or 250 rads per day. The survival is highly significantly better (p < .005) with the larger daily increments. There was a slight increase in acute symp-

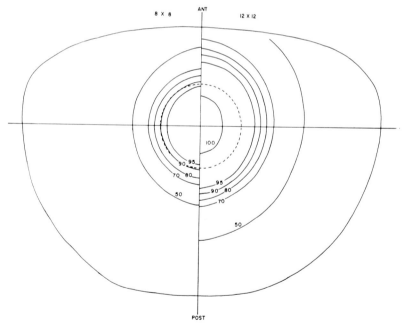

FIGURE 6-5B. 360° rotation with 8 × 8 cm field on the left and 12 × 12 cm field on the right ($^{60}$cobalt) .

TABLE 6-III

INFLUENCE OF DAILY DOSE ON REACTION (FINNEY)[96]

| Daily Tumor Dose (rads) (35 cases/group) | Rectal Reactions Acute Reactions | Chronic Reactions | Urodynia Symptom Improved | Symptom Unchanged | Symptom Deteriorated |
|---|---|---|---|---|---|
| 200 | 3 | — | 7 | 14 | 14 |
| 300 | 25 | 5 | 3 | 20 | 12 |

tomatology in those treated more rapidly and a small increase in chronic reactions in the same group. Table 6-III shows that the influence of daily tumor dose on rectal reactions was more important than on the urinary symptoms. Finney's[97] patients are now being treated with a four-field technique in an effort to spare the rectum more than is possible with even a three-field technique. With four-field or rotational therapy one would

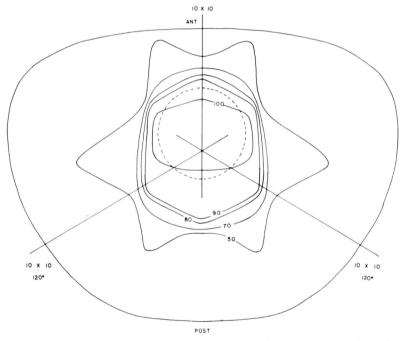

FIGURE 6-6. Three-field technique with 26 mvp betatron x-rays. The dose pattern is superior to even that shown in Figure 6-3.

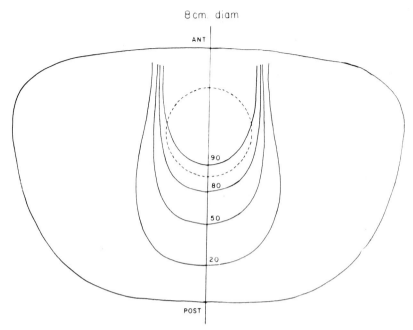

8 cm. diam

ANT

90

80

50

20

POST

FIGURE 6-7. Dose distribution with a single anterior 26 mev betatron electron beam. A large volume anterior is treated to a high dose, but there is sparing posteriorly.

anticipate rectal reactions would be minimized even with daily tumor doses of 300 rads.

Split-course therapy perhaps is a method of reducing the incidence of normal tissue reactions, yet still obtaining a satisfactory control rate of the primary tumor.[133, 240, 242] With this treatment regimen, a dose of 3,000 rads in 2 weeks (10 treatments) may be given followed by a rest period of 3 to 3½ weeks. Treatment is then resumed with another 3,000 rads in 2 weeks if there is no evidence of spread or deterioration in the patient's general condition. Treatment by this technique, using large portals, necessitates protraction of each treatment course for 2½ weeks (12 treatments) with a similar interval between courses. Supplemental local treatment can be given at the end of such a split-course if deemed advisable.

Irradiation with patients in hyperbaric oxygen atmosphere has been utilized in an attempt to improve local curability of bladder tumors. Most malignant tumors have hypoxic cells and these are less sensitive to irradiation than well oxygenated cells. If these hypoxic cells could be made better oxygenated, then their sensitivity to irradiation would be increased considerably while effecting little the sensitivity of previously well oxygenated cells, for example, those in normal tissues. No well-controlled studies have been completed, but there is a recent in progress report by Cade and McEwen[46] of St. Mary's Hospital in Portsmouth, England; randomized patients were treated to doses of 6,000 rads in eight weeks using five treatments per week. Forty patients with bladder carcinoma had been included in the study at the time of the report; all had been followed for at least six months. Thirteen of the patients treated in air survived whereas only eight patients treated in hyperbaric oxygen were living. Distant metastases were noted in three patients treated in air and in six patients treated in hyperbaric oxygen. A review of the randomized series indicates a case selection against the oxygen series in that of eight patients in the entire group with unfavorable squamous cell carcinomas or anaplastic carcinomas, seven were included in the hyperbaric oxygen grouping. Also, there were more Stage C lesions in the hyperbaric oxygen group. Total doses utilized were somewhat less than most radiotherapists would advise. It may be that the real advantage of irradiation in hyperbaric oxygen will be in the early lesions, either patients with multiple Stage A tumors or Stage $B_1$ lesions.

Local hyperthermia ultimately may prove beneficial in improving the therapeutic index in bladder tumors. Only a preliminary experimental report is included in the literature.[53]

Brizel and Scott[36] have suggested a rapid palliative approach to patients with Stage D disease and their results in a small group of patients is surprisingly good with doses of 3,500 R in 11 treatments over 14 elapsed days. Of the patients treated since July, 1962, 8 of 17 survived one year after treatment and 2 of 6, three years or more after treatment. The palliative role of radiotherapy has been considered by others using different techniques.[60, 123, 205, 217]

The major problem associated with external irradiation is

radiation cystitis which manifests itself clinically with urodynia and increased frequency.[19] Bleeding may be seen in the more severe cases. The symptoms are usually more frequent and serious in patients with multiple prior surgical procedures, particularly patients who have had segmental resection or cystotomy.[18, 48, 54, 62, 100] Patients who are asymptomatic, except for hematuria, at the start of irradiation ordinarily tolerate treatment very well and are unlikely to have any long term morbidity. In contrast, however, patients with symptoms at the start of treatment may have increased symptomatology during the course of irradiation and may have some long term morbidity, ordinarily increased frequency and occasionally urodynia.

Hemorrhagic radiation cystitis is occasionally seen.[116] It is an advanced, chronic reaction to irradiation and may become clinically apparent from several months to several years or longer after radiotherapy. The mucosa is atrophic, edematous, thin, and pale; the submucosa is fibrotic and capillary dilatation is seen. Contractibility of the involved vessels is impaired since the arteriolar musculature is replaced by fibrous tissue. These alterations can be the source of recurrent, often profuse, hemorrhage. Conservative management is apparently the most successful approach, although not entirely satisfactory in some cases. Cortisone or cortisone derivatives may help decrease the inflammatory reaction and arteriolitis. Irrigations of the bladder with saline, silver nitrate solution, or 6-aminocaproic acid have been helpful in selected cases. Appropriate blood replacement is beneficial. Fulguration of telangiectatic areas is hazardous since necrotic ulcers or fistulae may be produced; bleeding is controlled infrequently by this approach unless a specific bleeding point is identified. Urinary diversion may be necessary in cases not responding to conservative management. Bilateral hypogastric artery ligation also is thought beneficial. Cystectomy may be required in the recalcitrant cases.

Careful attention to radiotherapeutic techniques and control of urinary symptomatology during a course of irradiation minimizes the frequency of post irradiation cystitis. It is necessary to attempt to control urinary infection before and during treatment. After an operative procedure on the bladder, an interval of at least three weeks prior to initiation of radiotherapy is advised. This allows a reasonable period for the mucosa to heal and for antibiotic therapy to clear any infection secondary to the operation.

During treatment, a patient with urodynia and frequency is placed on a bladder sedative, given a broad-spectrum antibiotic (after obtaining a urine culture), started on analgesics, and instructed to maintain a good fluid intake during the day, restricting this after approximately 6 PM. It is not advisable to catheterize these patients during radiotherapy or in the first several weeks following conclusion of irradiation, since this may be instrumental in causing a chronic postirradiation urethral obstruction. If there is urethral or bladder neck obstruction, a cystotomy tube may be preferable to an indwelling urethral catheter. However, it is preferable to keep all tubes out of the bladder unless absolutely essential since secondary infection and mucosal irritation so frequently result.

Ascending urinary tract infection is seen occasionally during a course of radiotherapy. This most frequently occurs in patients with ureterovesical obstruction and cystitis. It is often a fatal complication and must be treated vigorously.[84, 198] Specific antibiotic therapy usually is sufficient; in some instances it is necessary to do a ureteral diversion.

Recto-sigmoiditis may be seen either acutely or subsequent to conclusion of a course of radiotherapy.[86, 234] This is seen most frequently in patients who have disease extending into the prostate; in these instances it is necessary, of course, to deliver a cancericidal dose to the anterior wall of the rectum. Significant sigmoiditis is more frequent in patients with colonic diverticula.

For sigmoiditis occurring during the course of irradiation, paregoric or Lomotil® is prescribed. The patients are asked to restrict their intake of fresh fruits and vegetables and other incompletely digestable food. If diarrhea does not subside on this regimen or if there is bloody diarrhea, then the treatment must be interrupted, resuming cautiously after subsidence of signs and symptoms.

The diarrhea and cramping may persist in some patients following conclusion of treatment or clinical subacute or chronic sigmoiditis may develop after a latent period of several months (rarely years). Diet is important since irritation of the bowel must be minimized. Mineral oil may be used to keep the stools soft. Cortisone enemas (25-50 mg prednisolone acetate/50 ml water everyday) may be helpful in some cases. Rarely a diverting colostomy will be necessary; patients requiring this procedure will ordinarily have severe reactions, usually with frequent, bloody diarrhea.

Small bowel complications are very rare.[86] Small bowel stenosis or fistulae do occur, however, particularly is there has been prior abdominal surgery. In such a situation, there are usually postoperative adhesions which restrict the mobility of the bowel; as a consequence a fixed loop of small bowel may be repeatedly irradiated during the course of treatment.

Resection of involved segments is required infrequently; often healing is delayed and anastomotic leaks develop. Good margins of apparently normal bowel at the site of anastomosis reduce the frequency of subsequent fistulae.

Short-term morbidity (diarrhea and/or cystitis usually) of varying severity is seen in most patients treated to cancericidal doses. The symptoms ordinarily gradually decrease in significance about 10 days following conclusion of irradiation and by 3 weeks post-treatment the majority of patients are essentially well. Three to 10 per cent of patients alive one year after treatment may have moderate or severe morbidity, usually secondary to cystitis;[48] this is less than the operative mortality rate of cystectomy.

Busby[43] treated 44 patients with carcinoma of the bladder with [60]cobalt doses of 5,000 to 7,000 rads in three to six weeks. Nineteen patients are alive, 12 free of tumor for varying periods. The referring physicians were contacted regarding their feelings about 18 of the surviving patients; they considered the results good in 15 and fair in 3. When asked "if faced with a similar problem, would you recommend cobalt therapy?" the same physicians responded affirmatively in 17 instances and there was only a single negative reply. Sixteen of the 18 patients were contacted. Eleven thought their responses had been good with the others acknowledging a fair response. Fourteen of the

16 patients would accept cobalt therapy "if faced with the same problem again."

Patients should not be cystoscoped until at least three months following irradiation so as not to aggravate any irradiation reactions still present. Cystoscopy is always associated with the risk of infection and this risk is increased in the post-irradiation period. Cystoscopic evaluation is difficult during the immediate post-irradiation period for it is often impossible to distinguish between tumor and reaction. Biopsies done before three months may be misleading for some bladder tumors regress very slowly and a positive biopsy less than three months following conclusion of irradiation is ordinarily not significant. Some patients have been "cured" by biopsy alone three to six months following irradiation.

Patients must be followed at least every three months after conclusion of irradiation so that resectable, persistent tumor can be dealt with promptly. A transurethral resection will occasionally cure a small residual tumor, particularly in patients initially having Stage A or $B_1$ tumors.

Occasionally, cystectomy is required after irradiation.[129, 274] If moderate field therapy has been used, the complication rate for cystectomy is not much higher than in patients not previously irradiated.[294] Cystectomy may be necessary for persistent local tumor; as many as 25 per cent of patients with persistent tumor in the bladder may be salvaged by post irradiation cystectomy. Thirty-three per cent of Whitmore's cases with superficial tumors, previously irradiated to approximately 6,000 rads in six weeks, survived following cystectomy for persistence.[294] Similar results may hold for selected patients treated for deeply infiltrating tumors who show local persistence post irradiation but are thought suitable for resection. Rarely, cystectomy also may be necessary in patients without evidence of persistent tumor for either contracture or unremitting hemorrhagic cystitis post irradiation.

## B. Intracavitary Radiation

Papillomas of the bladder and some Stage A tumors, particularly if multiple, may be difficult to control with resection or fulguration through a cystoscope or even at open cystotomy. In such situations, radioactive materials have been instilled into the bladder or in rubber balloon catheters in an effort to achieve tumoricidal doses to the mucosa with relative sparing of the submucosa and muscular layers of the bladder. These techniques have now been in use for 12 to 15 years in some centers; the indications and results of this form of irradiation are becoming better defined.

The most commonly used isotope is colloidal [198]gold which has a half life of 2.7 days and emits .96 mev beta particles and a spectrum of gamma rays. The beta emission is responsible for the majority of the irradiation at the surface amounting to approximately 90 per cent of the dose. But the beta rays have limited penetration; e.g. the dose at a depth of 0.3 mm is half of the dose at the surface (half value depth of 0.3 mm).[89, 172, 263] Some superficial tumors are considerably thicker than 0.3 mm, of course.

Three hundred millicuries of colloidal [198]gold, diluted in 100 milliliters of saline, are instilled into the bladder after introduction of a Foley catheter and inflation of a catheter balloon.[76, 263] After $2\frac{1}{2}$ hours, the bladder contents are drained and the bladder washed eight times in saline. This gives a calculated surface dose of 3,000 R. The treatment is repeated ordinarily after six to eight weeks. Ellis[90] has prepared a nomograph to assist in calculating doses depending on the volume of solution and the number of millicuries of [198]gold used. The proximal urethra will not be adequately irradiated by this approach, so he has suggested using [60]cobalt in a balloon introduced via a perineal urethrotomy as well.

Several problems are associated with using [198]gold for treatment in addition to the radiation hazard.[76, 90] Cystitis with bladder contraction has been seen in many of the patients who have been irradiated sufficiently to control their papillomas. Ulceration of the bladder mucosa is occasionally seen.

[111]Silver, [32]phosphorus, [90]yttrium, and [76]arsenic also have been instilled into the bladder.[87, 89, 202, 272, 301] The half value depths for these isotopes are 0.4 mm, 0.8 mm, 1.0 mm, and 1.3 mm, respectively (Fig. 6-8). With the more penetrating beta rays, it

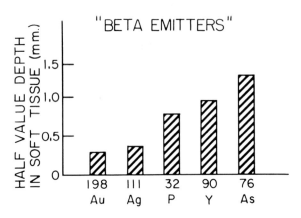

Figure 6-8. Depth of penetration for "beta emitters." The half value layer is the thickness of soft tissue which reduces the dose to 50 per cent of the mucosal or maximal dose. "Beta emitters" have either negligible or no gamma emissions.

was hoped that a better tumor control rate could be achieved; this has not definitely been established, however. Einhorn and associates,[87] using [76]As, noted that with surface doses of 6,300 to 6,700 R over 15 to 22 days, papillomas persisted in all three patients so treated. Papillomas also persisted in three out of eight patients treated with doses of 7,000 to 10,500 R over 13 to 34 days. In four others of the latter group, there was subsequent recurrence after intervals of 9 to 21 months. Recurrences after fulguration were less frequent than before radiotherapy in all patients, however.

Moreover, of considerable concern was the severe bladder contraction seen. All patients with doses in excess of 8,200 R to the mucosal surface required cystectomies during the second year postirradiation because of marked hemorrhage. Histologic examinations of these bladders showed marked fibrosis which extended through the bladder wall into the perivesical fat. Telangectasia of the mucosa and the submucosa tended to increase with the dose used. Ulceration and necrosis of the mucosal surface was noted in two of five patients requiring cystectomy. There was edema throughout the bladder wall in most cases. Vesico-ureteral reflex was also common after treatment with intravesical [76]arsenic, appearing in eight out of nine patients treated by Einhorn and associates.[87]

Papillomata also have been treated with gamma emitting isotopes, either as a solution ([82]bromine, [24]sodium, or [60]cobalt, e.g.) or a solid source within an intravesical balloon.[172, 209, 282] The instillation method is suitable for treating lesions which are more deeply infiltrating than those which can be irradiated with beta emitters. Nevertheless, the dose at a depth of 15 mm from this technique is no more than 50 per cent of the maximum and consequently tumors which infiltrate into the deep muscle or extend into the perivesical fat are inadequately irradiated. Complications of contraction, hemorrhagic cystitis, and calculi occur in at least 20 per cent of treated patients.

Friedman[107, 108] has had fantastic results in treating patients with intracavitary radium or [60]cobalt in the center of a 30 cc intravesical balloon inflated to the shape of a sphere or spheroid. The balloon is placed at cystotomy. The central source is approximately 2.2 cm from the surface; the source strength is such that it delivers a surface dose of 1,000 rads per day. Careful attention to the details of treatment is essential. An appropriate balloon must be selected to irradiate uniformly the lower three-fifths of the bladder. The position of the source is verified frequently during the course of treatment. Two placements are usually required. The first is to a mucosal dose of 4,000 rads in 4 days; 7 to 10 days later another placement is made. Friedman tailors the dose of this second placement according to the findings after the initial treatment. A tumor which has markedly shrunk may be treated to only an additional 2,000 rads, whereas one with minimal regression may be given as much as 6,000 rads more.

Friedman[109] reported in 1958 the results of 34 patients followed for more than five years. Eighty-five per cent of operative Stage O, A, or $B_1$ tumors were controlled as were 47 per cent of Stage $B_2$ and C lesions. These results were not updated in a 1968 paper.[107] The results of Sell[248] are not quite so good, but he was dealing with a more advanced group of patients, many of whom had major resections prior to radiotherapy. Seventeen of 50 patients he treated with intracavitary radium were alive after an observation period of five years. Only 5 of 16 cases with malignant bladder tumors treated by Bratherton[33] by this method were alive and well at 2 years after treatment.

*sixty-seven*

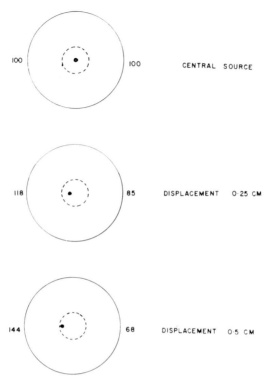

FIGURE 6-9. Effect of asymmetrical placement of the [60]cobalt or radium source in the balloon catheter on mucosal dose.

Considerable experience is required to use intracavitary techniques, particularly the method introduced by Friedman. Asymmetrical placement of the central sources, even by as little as 5 mm, will cause a marked heterogeneity of dose. Figure 6-9 shows this graphically according to calculations made by Bratherton.[33] Contraindications for use of a central radioactive source include previous irradiation, tumors of the dome, bladder capacity below 100 cc, grossly palpable tumor (tumor thicker than 2.5 cm), urethral stricture, poor general condition, *or in any case suitable for interstitial implantation.*[107]

Intracavitary techniques are associated with higher rates of complications than seen following external radiotherapy. Since it now is possible to treat carcinomas of the bladder with external megavoltage beams, there is less need to utilize these intracavitary techniques. If all operators had the success of Friedman,[109] this would not be an appropriate conclusion. However, others have not been able to use this method with the same degree of effectiveness.[56, 126, 130, 248] Lougheed[171] suggests using this approach in combination with external beam irradiation.

## C. Interstitial Irradiation

Direct implantation of bladder tumors with radioactive sources has been used for more than 50 years.[10, 11, 63, 91, 197, 234, 260] In 1942, Barringer[11] reported on 257 of his own cases of bladder cancers seen before 1937. These patients were treated with radon seed implantation following fulguration. In a fourth of the cases, the implantation was accomplished through the cystoscope. In the other three-fourths, the implant was accomplished at the time of suprapubic cystotomy. Patients at that time who had widely disseminated papillomata or papillary carcinoma were treated by cystectomy and infiltrating lesions arising in the bladder vault were excised. The other papillary

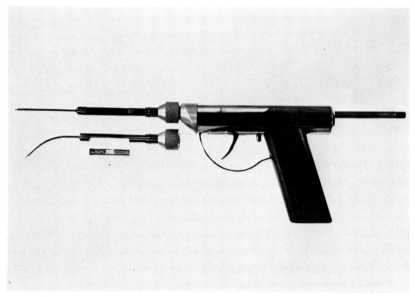

FIGURE 6-10A. The Royal Marsden gold grain gun and cartridge.

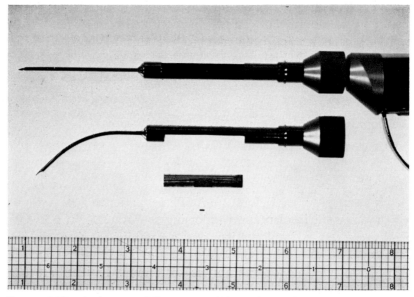

FIGURE 6-10B. A close-up of the gun, straight and curved implanters, cartridge, and a grain. Scale in inches.

and infiltrating tumors were implanted following resection or fulguration. Fifty-six per cent of the patients with papillary cancers were well at five years and 29 per cent with infiltrating cancers were well a similar length of time; 32 patients who died of intercurrent disease or were lost to follow up were excluded, as were 15 cases treated palliatively. Complications subsequent to treatment included cystitis and urinary bladder stone formation.

Recently, [198]gold grains have been used as a radon seed substitute to treat localized bladder tumors through a cystotomy following resection or fulguration.[215, 234] The gold grains are inserted in the tumor base with a gold grain gun;[131] the gun is shown in Figures 6-10A and 6-10B. Cartridges containing 14 gold grains allow rapid implantation. Distribution of the gold grains is according to rules that have been established. A 4 to 5 cm diameter tumor is the largest which can be effectively implanted. The gold grains are now available in this country from several suppliers at reasonable cost. [51]Chromium, producing

*seventy*

low energy gamma rays, may also be used by the same method. Figure 6-11 shows a bladder tumor implanted with [198]gold grains. Poole-Wilson[221] indicates that results from this approach are better than Marshall has reported in selected patients treated by segmental resection.

Radium implants also have been used with considerable effectiveness in recent years.[138, 167] Van der Werf-Messing[285] treated 148 cases of histologically confirmed carcinomas of the bladder between 1951 and 1959 with radium. The needles were implanted during suprapubic cystectomy. Table 6-IV shows the relationship between stage and curability by this tech-

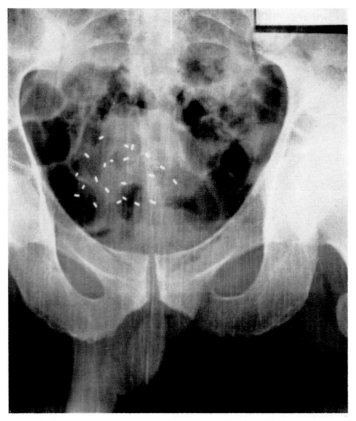

FIGURE 6-11. X-ray of the bladder showing [198]gold grains in place. Implant of base of papillary tumor followed resection at cystotomy.

TABLE 6-IV

## RESULTS OF INTRACAVITY OR INTERSTITIAL
### IRRADIATION (5 YR. SURVIVAL)

| Operative Stage | St. O, A, B, or $T_1$ Per Cent | St. $B_2$, C or $T_2$, $T_3$ Per Cent | St. D Per Cent |
|---|---|---|---|
| 1) Friedman (central intracavitary radium— 34 pts.)[109] | 85 | 47 | 0 |
| 2) Bloom (tantalum implant—75 pts.)[21] | 70 | 40 | — |
| 3) Van der Werf-Messing (radium implant— 148 pts.)[285] | 64 | 26 | — |

nique as well as by other interstitial approaches. Others not included in the table also have used radium and other sources effectively.[271, 277]

[182]Tantalum wire is suitable for selected cases, usually in patients with a large solitary tumor which may be infiltrating muscle.[21, 265, 281] Figure 6-12 shows a tantalum wire inducer and hair pin wire. The half life of [182]tantalum is 111 days, which means that the pins can be kept in stock and consequently are available as needed. Figure 6-13 shows the technique whereby implantation is accomplished and Figure 6-14 shows a [182]tantalum implant. The wire is attached to a thread which is

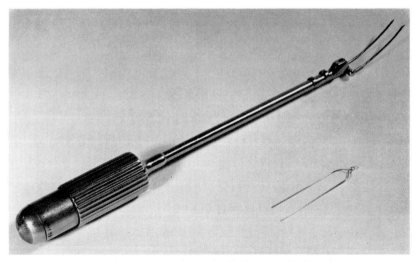

FIGURE 6-12. [182]tantalum wire inducer and wire pin.

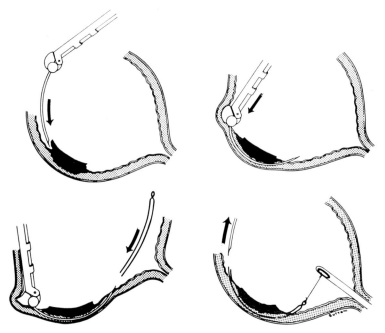

FIGURE 6-13. Technique for inserting the [182]tantalum wire pin.

brought out through the urethra after implantation. It is thereby possible to remove the tantalum wire transurethrally after the desired time for implant, which is usually of the order of five to seven days. The plan ordinarily is to deliver 6,000 to 6,500 R at 0.5 cm from the plane of the implant.

Bloom (and Wallace)[21] reported on their results with 250 cases treated with [182]tantalum in 1960. Of the $T_1$ lesions, 70 per cent survived at five years and of the $T_2$ lesions, 40 per cent survived at five years. Their complication rate was low. Total cystectomy was carried out in 8 per cent of the patients for residual tumor, a new tumor, or for radio-necrosis mistaken for tumor. Bloom intends to update his experience for presentation in the near future; his present results, nevertheless, approximate those reported in 1960. The technique requires extreme cooperation between the urologist and radiotherapist. Such cooperation, however, results in a satisfactory cure rate in suitable patients.

The complication rate with interstitial therapy is less serious

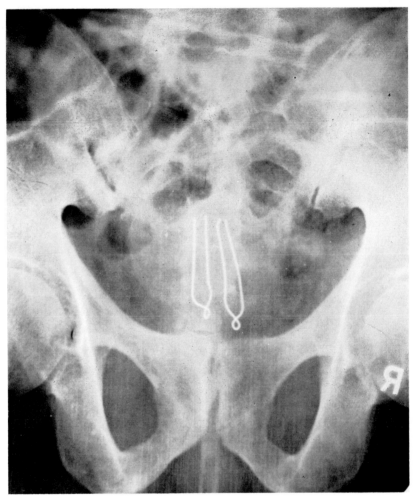

FIGURE 6-14. X-ray of [182]tantalum wire implant. This type of implant is useful for broad-based sessile tumors which are solitary and extend no deeper than the muscle.

than following intracavitary therapy, but postirradiation cystitis, bladder calculi, bladder contraction, and hemorrhage may be seen. Fistula formation also has been reported. This is a technique which has been used too infrequently in this country and perhaps reflects the lack of satisfactory working arrangements between most urologists and radiotherapists.

*Chapter 7*

# Operative Procedures

SINCE most patients with carcinoma of the bladder are initially seen for diagnostic evaluation by a urologist, perhaps it is not surprising that most bladder tumors are treated by some operative technique. The operative procedure may be resection or fulguration through a resectoscope or at cystotomy, segmental resection, or either simple or radical cystectomy. Denudation of bladder epithelium is a technique of rather recent origin, useful perhaps in the management of certain Stage O and A lesions; the long-term results and possible complications from this technique are not as yet appreciated.[7, 80, 125]

Deep resection or fulguration (transurethral resection) is effective in controlling low grade, Stage A tumors and a rare Stage $B_1$ tumor of low grade malignancy.[9, 13, 17, 31, 83, 186, 200, 201, 211, 212, 224, 275] Papillomas, if not too numerous, also can be controlled by this conservative approach. Nichols and Marshall[211] reported an 80 per cent survival of Stage O and A lesions, but only 3 of 18 cases with Stage B and C lesions were controlled by this method. Barnes[9] reported a 61 per cent (144/227) five-year survival for patients with Stage O and A lesions, and a 41 per cent (45/111) survival for those with Stage $B_1$ or $B_2$ tumors treated endoscopically. In some instances, because of site of origin or multiplicity of tumors, cystotomy is necessary for resection of localized tumors. However, open cystotomy is done only on indication since tumor implants in the bladder and abdominal wall incisions are not infrequently seen subsequently. Contraindications to local resection or fulguration include poorly differentiated cancer, invasion of the deep musculature, rapid recurrences of multiple, extensive tumors, or invasion of the prostate.[142]

Thompson and Kaplan[259] have described the resection procedure clearly. "The surgeon must depend chiefly on the gross differences in tissue appearance throughout his resection. In most cases, the border of the tumor is well defined and its homogeneous gelatinous character, coupled with its slightly yellow or gray color, contrasts sufficiently with the muscle to provide a reliable guide as to depth and extent of operation. Finally, the interlacing bundles of muscle can easily be recognized and it seems that no malignant tissue remains. At this stage, additional pieces of tissue are excised from the periphery and depth of the area and examined by frozen tissue methods. If these are negative, the operation is completed. If, however, the tissue is positive, additional strips can be excised until obviously perivesical tissue, including fat, is obtained by the excursion of the loop. At this point, one must be careful not to overdistend the bladder or extravasation of a serious degree can result. If tumor cells have penetrated the bladder wall, it seems logical that radiation must provide whatever additional curative measures are possible."

Segmental resection has been utilized in Stage A, Stage $B_1$ and $B_2$ and an occasional Stage C tumor.[31, 122, 139, 140, 141, 145, 179, 186, 189, 200, 224, 232, 275] This method of treatment is only applicable to tumors which are solitary and arise in the vault of the bladder. Since there are numerous circumferential lymphatics in the bladder wall, some therapeutic compromise may be associated with limited resection, especially for the more malignant tumors which are infiltrating into deep muscle or beyond. A 2 cm margin about the tumor is the minimal allowable clearance. Figure 7-1 shows an operative specimen from a patient who had an extensive segmental resection. Masina,[189] a proponent of this method, imagines

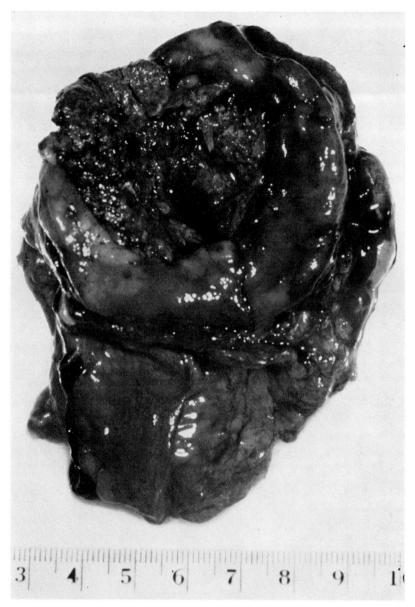

FIGURE 7-1. An extensive segmental resection specimen showing a high grade, infiltrating transitional cell carcinoma. Histology shown in Fig. 4-3A.

TABLE 7-I

PARTIAL CYSTECTOMY (5 YR. SURVIVAL)

| Operative Stage | St. O, A, B, or $T_1$ Per Cent | St. $B_2$, C, or $T_2$, $T_3$ Per Cent |
|---|---|---|
| Masina (58 pts.)[189] | 50 | 33 |
| Riches (59 pts.)[233] | 50 | 30 |
| Magri (45 pts.)[179] | 80 | 33 |
| Jewett (133 pts.)[141] | 58 | 16 |
| Marshall (123 pts.)[188] | 65 | 29 |

TABLE 7-II

CYSTECTOMY (5 YEAR SURVIVAL)

| Surgical Stage | St. O, A, $B_1$ or $T_1$ Per Cent | St. $B_2$, C or $T_2$, $T_3$ Per Cent | St. D Per Cent |
|---|---|---|---|
| Stone (37 pts.)[255] | 80 | 36 | 12 |
| Cordonnier (99 pts.)[58] | 52 | 33 | 0 |
| Whitmore and Marshall (230 pts.)*[290] | 47 | 14 | 0 |
| Glantz (36 pts.)[114] | 45 | 8 | 0 |
| Jewett, King, and Shelley (71 pts.)[145] | 38 | 13 | 0 |
| Riches (77 pts.)[233] | 32 | 8 | 0 |

* Ten-year survival 29 per cent for Stage O, A, $B_1$; 40 per cent when corrected for natural attrition. 8.5 per cent for Stage $B_2$, C; 12 per cent when corrected for natural attrition.

that less than 5 per cent of patients with tumors of the bladder can be satisfactorily managed by this approach. Marshall[188] treated 12 per cent of his large series of bladder cancers with segmental resections. In the patients with well defined lesions, without mucosal changes elsewhere in the bladder, good results can be obtained. Masina[189] reported 81 per cent (13/16) five-year survival in such $T_1$ lesions. The results of others' experiences with partial cystectomy are indicated in Table 7-I. All cases were staged at operation.

Cystectomy with urinary diversion has been used in the treatment of bladder tumors for several decades.[13, 26, 27, 31, 34, 58, 59, 122, 139, 140, 141, 186, 223, 224, 232–234, 255, 274, 275, 290] Although theoretically a valid approach, cystectomy has not resulted in the cure rates which might have been expected. This is particularly so for operative Stage $B_2$ and C lesions. Presumably the presence of pelvic lymph nodes in more than 50 per cent of these patients is the major factor responsible for the poor results. Dissemination of tumor by operative manipulation also must play a role. Survival in patients treated by this method is indicated in Table 7-II; cures range from the 36 per cent of Stone[255] to the 8 per cent of Riches[233] and of Glantz.[114] Of 218 patients with Grade 2 or above bladder tumors seen at the Bladder Tumor Registry from 1931 to 1951, there were 37 (17 per cent) alive and well at 3 years following total cystectomy; sixteen other cases died in the next $1\frac{1}{2}$ years.[245]

Cordonnier[59] believes the indications for cystectomy are as follows: "1) All lesions which show definite muscle invasion; 2) rapidly recurring Grade II lesions showing a tendency to increased cellular malignancy and apparently out of control on management by conservative means, and 3) all sessile Grade III and IV lesions." Unless obviously inoperable, all patients with advanced carcinoma are explored since it is impossible to accurately assess operability prior to surgery.

With simple total cystectomy, the bladder, prostate, seminal vesicles, and some of the perivesical lymph nodes and a portion of the pelvic peritoneum are removed. In all females, the entire urethra should be removed at the time of cystectomy and likewise, the urethra should be removed in all males who show multicentric papillary tumors. A total cystectomy specimen with transitional cell carcinoma is shown in Figures 7-2A and 7-2B. Radical cystectomy is intended to clear the pelvis of all its contents with the exception of the rectum. The pelvic peritoneum and all lymph nodes medial and lateral to the external iliac vessels from the bifurcation of the aorta to the femoral canal are removed. In women, the operation also includes removal of the uterus, ovaries, broad ligaments, and anterior wall of the vagina.[147, 294]

Radical cystectomy undoubtedly adds little to the survival rate possible with total cystectomy. Most urologists feel that if the lymph nodes are clinically positive, even a cystectomy is not indicated since only a very rare case might be expected to be

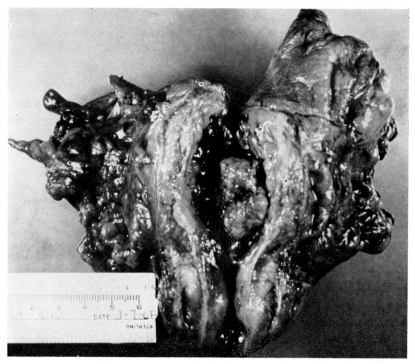

FIGURE 7-2A. A total cystectomy specimen.

cured.[114, 140] The value of a pelvic node dissection, a less than ideal operative procedure at best, in patients with clinically latent metastases is uncertain. Apparently, few patients with no more than microscopic lymph node metastases are cured by even a radical procedure. Wallace,[277] with his vast experience, has only one five-year survivor among all patients with histologically proven lymph node metastases treated by radical cystectomy.

MacKenzie and Whitmore[173] reported in 1968 on their results in five patients with bladder cancer treated with a supraradical cystectomy; all four pubic rami were removed for tumor in the retro pubic space. Two of the patients were alive in 1967; one, however, was resected in August 1966, and the other required a translumbar amputation for persistence 6 months after resection of the pubic rami in conjunction with pelvic exenteration.

Comparison of treatment results in patients (not randomized and with selection probably favoring the segmental resection group) with bladder cancer managed either by segmental resection or cystectomy is shown in Tables 7-IIIa and 7-IIIb. Long term renal complication subsequent to urinary diversion adversely affected the survival statistics of the cystectomy series. In recent years, these problems have become somewhat less frequent, but Brunschwig and Barber[40] reported in 1968 that in those who live more than five years after pelvic exenteration for advanced cancer, the most frequent cause of death was uremia or urinary tract sepsis. Once urinary diversion is done, constant observation is necessary to detect evidence of progressing urinary tract dysfunction.[155, 169]

Cystectomy is associated with considerable mortality even

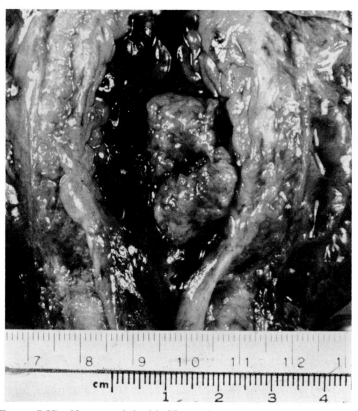

FIGURE 7-2B. Close-up of the bladder and exophytic, ulcerated tumor.

TABLE 7-IIIa

SEGMENTAL RESECTION—133 CASES (JEWETT)[141]

| Stage | A & W 5 Yrs. | Died with Cancer | Died with Complications Late |
|---|---|---|---|
| A | 15/26 (58%) | 8/26 (31%) | 1/26 (4%) |
| B₁ | 7/12 (58%) | 5/12 (42%) | 0 |
| B₂ | 4/25 (16%) | 21/25 (84%) | 0 |
| C | 11/70 (16%) | 55/70 (78%) | 4/70 (6%) |
| | 37/133 | 89/133 | 5/133 |

TABLE 7-IIIb

TOTAL CYSTECTOMY—71 CASES (JEWETT)[141]

| Stage | A & W 5 Yrs. | Died with Cancer | Died with Renal Complications |
|---|---|---|---|
| A | 6/12 (50%) | 4/12 (33%) | 2/12 (17%) |
| B₁ | 2/4 | 1/4 | 1/4 |
| B₂ | 2/12 (16%) | 5/12 (42%) | 5/12 (42%) |
| C | 5/43 (12%) | 33/43 (77%) | 4/43 (9%) |
| | 15/71 | 43/71 | 12/71 |

when done by very experienced surgeons. Operative mortality ranges from 5 per cent (Bowles and Cordonnier[27]) to 14 per cent (Whitmore and Marshall[290]). Other significant postoperative complications (including wound infection, anastomotic leak, intestinal obstruction, and wound dehiscence) are seen in 12 to 25 per cent of patients. There are, of course, long term complications from urinary diversions as well. Numerous procedures (cutaneous ureterostomy, ureterosigmoidostomy, ileal loop diversion, etc.) have been developed to deal with the interrupted urinary tract, but none of the currently used methods are entirely acceptable.[16, 35, 124, 234, 262, 278, 279, 297] With an ileal loop, as many as 10 per cent of patients may develop significant upper urinary tract pathology; it is associated with fewer complications and less morbidity than other urinary diversions which have been used.[59, 65] Furthermore, improved appliances have made patient acceptance more satisfactory. A

*eighty-two*

recent leading article in the British Medical Journal succinctly summarizes the present status: "For the time being the ileal conduit remains the diversion, if not of choice at least of necessity."[164]

*Chapter 8*

---

# Chemotherapy

FOR more than 50 years, attempts have been made to eradicate bladder neoplasms by topical cytotoxic agents. Increasing strengths of silver nitrate were used initially by Herring[128] to treat vesical papillomas. Joseph reported on the use of trichloroacetic acid in 1919; Semple[249] in 1948 and Duckworth[82] in 1950 reported on their experience with podophyllin. Phenol and glycerin also have been used.

In 1958, Leroi and Leroi-von May[168] reported their experience with 15 patients with infiltrative bladder tumors treated with mistletoe extract. Nine patients had been followed for three years or more; six of these survived. All tumors were highly malignant and in several instances they were considered inoperable. The authors used an injectable mistletoe (Viscum album) preparation (from oak for men and from apple trees for women) mixed with "silver salts." This was administered in cycles of 14 injections starting with single low doses on alternate days, and then slowly increasing doses and dosage intervals. There is no other apparent reference in the literature to the use of this method and its rationale and mode of action certainly is not clear.

It was not until 1961, however, that a reasonably satisfactory agent was found; Jones and Swinney[146] reported on the use of the alkylating agent, thio-TEPA. Thirteen patients were treated by instilling thio-TEPA into the bladder. The usual dose decided upon after preliminary experience was obtained, was 90 mg dissolved in 50 ml of sterile water. The drug was retained in the bladder for three hours. Four instillations were used, usually at intervals of two to three days. There was almost complete disappearance of multiple papillary neoplasms in eight of the thirteen patients. Veenema and associates[266, 267, 270] and others[81, 146] also have reported on the use of thio-TEPA instilled into the bladder for carcinoma or papillomas. The follow-up interval has been short in all reported series. Wescott's[286] early impression was that thio-TEPA is effective in limiting the growth or activity of low grade, low stage bladder tumors and that it may be of benefit in preventing recurrences.

Esquivel, MacKenzie, and Whitmore[92] have used thio-TEPA, actinomycin D, and 5-fluorouracil in an effort to control bladder papillomas or various stages of bladder carcinoma. In three of eight patients with papillomas, there was complete disappearance of the tumor after an average of seven instillations (30 to 60 mg of thio-TEPA in 30 to 60 ml of water or saline per instillation) and two showed partial destruction of the tumor. Among seven patients with Stage B cancer, only one showed partial destruction of the tumor. One of four patients with papillomas treated with weekly instillations of 1.0 mg of actinomycin D and 30 ml of water or saline showed apparent necrotic changes in the tumor, but in none was disappearance or even decrease in size of a tumor observed. Weekly instillations of 5-fluorouracil (10 mg/kg of body weight in an equal volume of water or saline) were used in nine patients. In one patient, a papilloma showed partial destruction after the third instillation, but no destructive effects were noted in the tumors in the remaining eight patients.

Abbassian and Wallace[1] have found intravesical thio-TEPA effective in 8 of 13 patients treated by this method: three of these had complete regression and in five the regression was marked, but incomplete. Epodyl (1 gm in 100 ml of water at daily intervals for two weeks) was used in 15 patients. There were five complete regressions and three partial regressions. It is of interest that the tumors in the six female patients did not respond to either thio-TEPA or epodyl. Mannitol myleran in a dosage of 2 gm dissolved in 60 ml of water repeated on alternate days for 8 to 12 treatments resulted in partial regression in only 1 of 11 patients. Methotrexate (30 mg in 50 ml of water) instilled into the bladder daily for 12 consecutive days was ineffective in all three patients.

The use of intracavitary chemotherapy is associated with few of the complications seen with intracavitary radioactive solutions. However, this technique seems potentially worthwhile only in superficial lesions: certainly it is unreasonable to expect a surface application to be effective for infiltrating tumors. Also, for the superficial lesions, it will undoubtedly prove necessary to repeat the instillations for prolonged periods. Although often termed a prophylactic treatment, intracavitary chemotherapy can only be effective against established, viable, tumor cells. It may control clinically unrecognized disease, but unfortunately at this time no measures can prevent with certainty a new cancer from appearing in a susceptible bladder. True prophylaxis may be possible when the process of carcinogenesis becomes better understood.

Systemic 5-fluorouracil also has been used in an effort to palliate disseminated bladder cancer.[73] It has proven beneficial for short term palliation only in a few individuals. Prout and other coinvestigators[227] in an adjuvant clinical trial to evaluate the effectiveness of 5-fluorouracil in the treatment of invasive carcinoma of the bladder gave randomized patients either a placebo or 5-fluorouracil. The 5-fluorouracil was given intravenously, 15 mg/kg diluted in 500 ml of solution, over a 2 to 3 hour period for 5 consecutive days. Then 7.5 mg/kg was given every other day for a total of 60 days unless toxicity developed. Toxicity prompted interruption until correction of same. Ten of 14 tumors grew during the 60 day evaluation period when treated with 5-fluorouracil and 10 of 15 tumors grew while on a placebo; 6 tumors in each series more than doubled in size. Only 2 of the 5-fluorouracil treated tumors regressed, while 3 of the tumors which were not treated decreased in size. White blood cell depression ($<$4,000 cells/mm$^3$) was observed in only 2 of the 5-fluorouracil patients and in 1 of the control patients. The use of 5-fluorouracil systemically in conjunction with radiotherapy and operative procedures is discussed in Chapter 9. Other systemic cytotoxic agents currently in clinical use have been even less beneficial than 5-fluorouracil.

*Chapter 9*

# Combined Therapy

### A. Preoperative Irradiation Followed by Cystectomy

Because of the unsatisfactory survival rates reported in most series following cystectomy alone, there has been increasing interest in irradiating the bladder and perivesical tissues prior to cystectomy.[99, 122, 127, 163, 218, 225, 252, 287, 291, 294, 296] It is still too early to know whether this combined approach will increase the cure rate in patients with carcinoma of the bladder. Unfortunately, no randomized studies are in progress to test whether this approach is better than cystectomy alone or preferable to full dose external radiotherapy followed by cystectomy *only on indication* (persistent disease in the bladder three or more months following irradiation).

A sampling of results reported to date with preoperative irradiation are shown in Table 9-I. Galleher and associates[111, 112] have treated at least 33 patients with combined preoperative irradiation (4,500-6,600 rads/4½-6 wks.) and total cystectomy (1 to 42 months post irradiation). Nineteen patients had cystectomies within six months of conclusion of radiotherapy and 26 were resected within a year. Follow-up on these 33 patients extended from 10 to 81 months. Eight of 23 patients with tumor present

*eighty-eight*

## TABLE 9-I

### EXPERIENCES WITH PREOPERATIVE IRRADIATION AND CYSTECTOMY

| | Survival Rate | Follow-up Interval | Usual Preoperative Dose | Clinical Stages | |
| --- | --- | --- | --- | --- | --- |
| | | | | Stage O,A,B₁ | Stage B₂,C |
| Galleher, Young, Mowad, Wizenberg and Bloedorn[111] ............ | 5/12 4/9 | 3 yrs. 5 yrs. | 4,500 to 6,000 rads/5-6 wks. | 6/33 | 24/33 |
| Whitmore[288, 293] ................................ | 36% | 3 yrs. | 4,000 rads/4 wks. | 44/128 | 66/128 |
| Veenema, Guttman, Uson, Sagerman, Dean and Ciardullo[270] ....... | 35% | 1-5 yrs. | 3,000 to 4,000 rads/3-4 wks.* | 26/96 | 31/96 |
| DeWeerd and Colby[74] ...................... | 84% | 0-24 mo. (9/23 < 12 mo.) | 4,800/7 wks. (split course) | 11/23† | 10/23† |
| Stein and Kaufman[253] ..................... | 75% | 6-59 mo. | 3,500/3 wks. (+5Fu) | 12/24 | 12/24 |

Clinical Stages

* Some patients given supplemental postoperative irradiation.
† Pathologic Stage, ostirradiation.

in the cystectomy specimen were alive more than one year post resection; eight of ten patients with no apparent tumor in the cystectomy specimen survived one or more years following cystectomy. Complications included four operative deaths and seven instances of bowel fistulae. Bloedorn,[20] in an earlier review of the same series, commented that this combined approach is particularly rational for "that group of tumors in which the control of the disease is low when either form of treatment is used alone: large infiltrating tumors with palpable masses, tumors with extension outside the bladder (prostate, perivesical tissues, lymph nodes, and pelvic walls), all infiltrating squamous cell and adenocarcinomas, and multiple tumors with frequent recurrences or consecutive primaries."

Whitmore and associates[288, 293] reported in 1968 on 128 patients followed for three or more years following preoperative irradiation and subsequent radical cystectomy. The tumor dose preoperatively was 4,000 rads in four weeks given through opposed anterior and posterior portals measuring 10 × 10 or 10 × 12 cm. The three-year survival rate is compared by clinical stage in Table 9-II with the Stanford series treated with 6 mvp linear accelerator x rays.[48] The survival rate is similar. Only with the superficial tumors is there even an indication that preoperative irradiation and subsequent radical cystectomy is more beneficial than full dose radiotherapy with cystectomy only done on indication. It is the deep tumors (Stage $B_2$ and C) in which improvement in results were anticipated by the planned combined approach.

Radiotherapy, given preoperatively in Whitmore's series to a

TABLE 9-II

COMPARISON OF RESULTS AT THREE YEARS FOR PREOPERATIVE IRRADIATION AND CYSTECTOMY AND FOR IRRADIATION ALONE AS THE PRIMARY INITIAL THERAPY

| Clinical Stage | Whitmore[288, 293] Preoperative Irradiation Plus Radical Cystectomy (3-year Survival) | Caldwell and Associates[48] Irradiation Alone (3-year Survival) |
|---|---|---|
| O, A, $B_1$ | 26/44 (59%) | 19/38 (50%) |
| $B_2$, C | 19/66 (20%) | 24/77 (31%) |
| $D_1$ | 1/18 ( 6%) | 1/15 ( 7%) |

dose of only 4,000 rads in 4 weeks, was surprising in its effect on some bladder tumors. In the 44 clinical Stage O, A, or $B_1$ lesions, no tumor was found in 6 of the operative specimens and in 10 other cases there were *in situ* changes only. Nine of 79 clinical Stage $B_2$ or C cases had no tumors recognizable histologically in the resected tissue; 1 additional specimen showed *in situ* change only.

Mortality and morbidity with the combined approach was formidable, but not unlike that seen with cystectomy alone. Whitmore[294] reported an operative mortality of 12 per cent (vs 11 per cent without preoperative irradiation) and operative complications in another 43 per cent (vs 43 per cent for patients having radical cystectomy without prior irradiation). In patients requiring cystectomy following a complete, but unsuccessful, course of irradiation (usually (6,000 rads/5-6 wks.), the operative mortality increased slightly to 15 per cent and operative complications were seen in 54 per cent of the cases.

Veenema and associates[269] now have a five year experience in 109 patients treated with radiotherapy, surgery, and chemotherapy for carcinoma of the bladder; 93 patients had preoperative irradiation. Doses of 3,000 to 4,000 rads in three to four weeks were used with 3,000 rads being the usual dose. Two to four weeks following irradiation the patients were re-evaluated with cystoscopy, chest films, and an excretory urogram. If the lesion at that time was suitable for endoscopic resection (13 cases) or partial cystectomy (16 cases), then this procedure was performed. Otherwise, a total cystectomy (49 cases) was done. Fifteen patients were found nonresectable at operation following preoperative irradiation. Postoperative radiotherapy, with doses of 2,000 to 3,000 rads in two to three weeks was given following operation if there was evidence of extension of tumor outside of the bladder at the time of operation. In patients with Stage A tumors in whom the bladder was preserved, topical chemotherapy with thio-TEPA seemed beneficial, in conjunction with irradiation, to minimize recurrences in the bladder. Seventy-three per cent (19/26) of Stage A patients survived one to five years after therapy; survival rate was reduced to 45 per cent (14/35) for clinical Stage B cases, for the same follow-up interval. Two of 11 patients with Stage C tumor survived at one to five years, one with persistent tumor; there were no survivors of 25 Stage D patients.

More recently, Sagerman[239] has reviewed the cases from the Columbia University College of Physicians and Surgeons included in the preceding series. The results are similar. He suggests that further evaluation of combined treatment for invasive carcinoma should include cases given higher preoperative doses. Based on experience in 46 patients, Kaufman[147] became somewhat disenchanted with preoperative irradiation in doses of 5,500 rads or more. There were an "inordinate number of major complications." No enhancement of survival was realized either. A preoperative dose of about 3,500 rads in 3 weeks now is being used by Kaufman and his associates.[148] The optimum preoperative dose clearly is not known. Neither is the most advantageous time for operating postirradiation. And it may be, of course, that this approach does not contribute to the quantity and quality of survival at all.

In a preliminary communication, DeWeerd and Colby[74] reported their experience with 32 patients with bladder carcinoma treated by a planned program of combined radiotherapy and total or partial cystectomy and pelvic lymphadenectomy. A dose of 4,800 rads was given to the bladder and adjacent pelvic lymph nodes in two courses of 12 to 14 days separated by a rest interval of approximately 3 weeks. The patients have been followed a short time with only seven surviving 24 months or more. Twenty-seven of the patients, however, are still alive, 25 without evidence of cancer. Complications were frequent. Two patients died postoperatively.

Thompson[260] treated 21 patients with combined surgery and radiotherapy; these represented 30 per cent of his total of 70 patients. Stages of disease were not indicated, but presumably these were reasonably early lesions. None of the patients had cystectomy so his results are not included in Table 9-I. Patients were treated with open diathermic excision plus kilovoltage x ray therapy (5 patients), palliative ureteral transplantation plus kilovoltage x ray therapy (3 patients), open diathermic excision plus radium implant (2 patients), open diathermic excision plus radon implantation (6 patients), open diathermic excision plus external megavoltage radiotherapy (1 patient), and partial cystectomy plus wither radon seed implantation (2 patients) or kilovoltage x ray therapy (2 patients). In this heterogeneous group of patients, 2 of 8 survived 5 years, and 7 of 13 have survived 3 years.

Riches[234] reports a crude five-year survival of 14 per cent with preoperative irradiation followed by local excision or cystectomy, usually in patients thought unsuitable for partial cystectomy. He suggests the use of preirradiation urinary diversion to reduce the complications of preoperative irradiation. Hecker,[127] however, has experienced poor results with ileal loop diversion prior to radiotherapy.

After reviewing their series of 182 patients with bladder tumors treated in New Zealand from 1953 to 1962, Greenslade and associates[122] were concerned that treatment methods used (primarily operative) had yielded discouraging results. They indicated an intention to use preoperative radiotherapy and surgery more frequently in patients suitable for an attempt at cure; their results from this approach should be forthcoming soon.

Wallace[278] suggests that preoperative radiotherapy permits assessment of tumors during a course of therapy. If a tumor is highly radiosensitive, then a full course is felt justified. If, however, at 4,000 rads there has been no response cystoscopically or on bimanual examination, a cystectomy is suggested. This is thought to give better comfort and perhaps even better survival than excessive irradiation of an insensitive tumor. Personally, I believe it is impossible to predict reliably the curability of any given tumor after doses of 4,000 rads. Certainly, some bladder tumors, cured by radiotherapy, may be very slow to regress.

Reports of long term results with the use of preoperative irradiation and subsequent cystectomy are being awaited anxiously. Present results do not show any startling improvement in survival. Since patients treated by this approach are committed to a cystectomy and urinary diversion by the combined program, I am loath to recommend it presently. Survival rates which are as satisfactory can undoubtedly be attained by doing cystectomies *only on indication* following a full course of radio-therapy. The major advantage of this suggested regimen is that many patients can keep their bladders and therefore need not contend with the morbidity (both psychologic and somatic) and mortality associated with urinary diversion.[47]

The method championed by Wallace[274] and Bloom[21] of using interstitial [198]gold or [182]tantalum in the base of selected Stage A and B tumors, following resection or fulguration at open cystectomy, is discussed in Chapter 6. Results from this combined approach are excellent and perhaps its use should be more widespread.

## B. Postoperative Irradiation

Postoperative irradiation should be reserved for treatment of patients found to have positive pelvic lymph nodes or invasion of perivesical structures at the time of cystectomy.[164] These Stage D patients are rarely cured, but worthwhile palliation (primarily prolongation of life) often is achieved.

Irradiation of the bladder also may be indicated following inadequate segmental resection or fulguration. In most cases, however, irradiation of this sort would be considered as the primary form of treatment rather than a supplement or complement to an operative approach. Volumes irradiated usually can be small, particularly if silver clips are placed at the margins of resection at operation.

## C. Combined Preoperative and Postoperative Irradiation

If, following preoperative irradiation, a tumor cannot be completely resected or there is pelvic adenopathy, it is probably advisable to give further irradiation postoperatively. This, of course, assumes that the preoperative dose is in the range of 3,000 to 4,000 rads and that the interval between conclusion of preoperative irradiation and availability for postoperative irradiation is no more than four to six weeks.

## D. Chemotherapy and Irradiation

As noted earlier, thio-TEPA intravesically has proven beneficial in selected cases with Stage O or Stage A tumors. Mechl and associates[191] have used intravesical thio-TEPA followed by irradiation in two groups of patients. The combined approach yielded favorable results in patients with papillomas, but the effects in patients with more advanced stage of neoplasm were no more than those after x-ray treatment alone.

Chemotherapy, primarily with 5-fluorouracil, also has been used in combination with radiotherapy in more advanced bladder tumors.[148, 150, 225, 227, 270] The 5-fluorouracil is given intravenously and radiotherapy is accomplished either subsequently or concomitantly. Early results from this combined approach have been forthcoming from several institutions. Woodruff, Murphy, and Hudson[298] used 5-fluorouracil and radiotherapy either as an adjuvant to an extirpative approach or as primary treatment where invasion precluded operative intervention. Fourteen patients with Stage B and C lesions were studied as well as 22 patients with Stage $D_1$ disease. Various techniques were used to administer the 5-fluorouracil. All patients, with one exception, received approximately 4,000 rads, tumor dose, with 2 mvp x rays. Approximately 50 per cent of the patients showed partial or complete tumor regression; the period of observation was less than a year in many of the patients.

Twenty-four patients have been treated with radiotherapy, chemotherapy and cystectomy by Stein and Kaufman.[253] 5-fluorouracil (initially total doses of 4 to 5 grams were used over 8 to 14 days; now 13 to 15 or more grams are given) and 3,500 rads (usual average tumor dose, $^{60}$cobalt) were given preoperatively for patients with Stage A through Stage C lesions. Additional patients with Stage D tumors, or those who were not suitable for operation, were treated with 5-fluorouracil (average total dose of 6 grams or more) and 5,500 rads tumor dose. Eleven of the Stage A to C patients had no demonstrable tumor in the resected specimen; this is surprising in view of the low doses of irradiation utilized. Eleven of the 12 patients with Stage A and $B_1$ lesions are alive and apparently well 10 to 14 months after initiation of treatment. Seven of the 12 cases with Stage $B_2$ and C disease are alive and well at 6 to 59 months. Seven patients, theoretically curable by extirpative operation, refused operation or were considered unsuitable surgical risks.

Four of these patients (treated by 5-fluorouracil and irradiation) were reported alive and well 10 or more months after initiation of treatment.

Morbidity with the combined approach was essentially unchanged from that seen with operation only. Suprapubic drainage persisted somewhat longer; now drains are not used at this site.[148] In 15 per cent of the cases, as a minimum, the stage of disease was reduced by the preoperative therapy.

The recent experiences with 5-fluorouracil in an ongoing adjuvant study to determine its effectiveness in the treatment of invasive carcinoma of the bladder gives little support to the contention that this agent is at all beneficial.[227] The details of this study are noted in Chapter 8. A placebo was as effective as 5-fluorouracil; in fact, in 14 paired patients, there was a better response with the placebo than with 5-fluorouracil. It may be, however, that 5-fluorouracil sensitizes a tumor to irradiation; further data are required to confirm this, however.

Burt, Kaufman and associates,[42] and Kaufman and Lichtenauer[149] have successfully transplanted human bladder cancer into the hampster cheek pouch in three instances. They are using the heterotransplanted tumors to evaluate the responsiveness to various chemotherapautic agents as well as irradiation. Mitomycin C, in doses acceptable for treatment in human subjects, showed the greatest effectiveness. One tumor was resistant to chemotherapy, but responsive to irradiation. A synergistic or potentiating action of irradiation and 5-fluorouracil in combination was demonstrated. Toxicity from a combined approach, however, may be severe. Immergut[136] has suggested, for example, that in clinical situations that irradiation be withheld always until toxic symptoms from systemic 5-fluorouracil cease. The optimum method of combining various treatment modalities has not been established. Test systems of this sort may prove beneficial in establishing the best therapeutic approach in selected patients with bladder neoplasms.

# Chapter 10

# Treatment Recommendations

THE lack of controlled treatment series has hampered therapeutic advances and undoubtedly has jeopardized the treatment of many patients. Such randomized clinical trials are imperative to allow valid evaluation of treatment results. For
clinical Stage $B_1$, $B_2$, and C lesions the results of cystectomy
alone, preoperative irradiation followed by cystectomy, and irradiation alone, with fulguration or cystectomy for persistent
disease only, should be evaluated; both quality and quantity of
survival should be studied. The patients irradiated only, could
be treated with a conventional uninterrupted course or with a
split-course regimen. In lieu of data from clinical trials, the following recommendations are made:

**Stage A:** Most Stage A tumors are low grade malignancies
and can be managed with deep, broad-based resection. If the
lesions are numerous, rapidly recurring, or other than low
grade lesions, radiotherapy is probably the treatment of choice.
For multiple lesions, the entire bladder should be irradiated
with doses of 6,000 to 6,500 rads in six weeks (four to five
treatments/week). Fields measuring $8 \times 8$ cm are usually adequate since the incidence of pelvic lymph node metastases is

*ninety-seven*

low. Treatment can be with a three field technique (two posterior obliques and an anterior field or two anterior obliques and a posterior field) or with 270° or 360° rotation. The patients must be very carefully followed postirradiation with cystoscopy at least every three months for the first two years post treatment and semiannually thereafter. Cystectomy, if feasible, is indicated for postirradiation recurrences, proven by biopsy three months or more after conclusion of irradiation.

Intravesical thio-TEPA may be valuable in controlling multiple superficial bladder tumors. This technique is a relatively new approach and long term results are not as yet known.

Some would use intracavitary irradiation, ordinarily a solid source in the center of a balloon catheter or a gamma emitting solution in an intravesical balloon, for treating Stage A lesions. These are specialized techniques and probably have no advantage over external radiotherapy with megavoltage beams. Significant discrepancies in doses predictably are frequent.

For the solitary, high grade Stage A lesions, local resection with $^{198}$gold grain implantation of the base of the tumor is perhaps the method of choice. Recurrences are less frequent than after resection alone.

**Stage $B_1$:** Clinical Stage $B_1$ tumors, particularly the high grade neoplasms, need aggressive therapy and should be treated with megavoltage radiations. They may be treated in the same fashion as indicated under Stage A, with multiple small fields or with rotational therapy.

Some may prefer using an intracavitary source and others might prefer interstitial implantation with $^{198}$gold grains, $^{182}$tantalum or radium rather than external radiotherapy. The $^{198}$gold grain technique is least cumbersome, but the volume which can be implanted with $^{198}$gold grains, however, is limited. All these implant methods necessitate a cystotomy. Although there are some risks to adjacent normal tissues from these techniques, they are less frequent and ordinarily less severe than following external radiotherapy.

Patients must be followed very closely postirradiation. Histologic proof of persistence, more than three months following conclusion of irradiation, is an indication for operative intervention, if feasible. Transurethral resection, segmental resection, or cystectomy can rescue some in whom there is persistent bladder neoplasm at the primary site following irradiation. Complications of resection are only minimally increased in the patients previously irradiated with small or moderate sized fields.[294]

Cystectomy has been advised for clinical Stage $B_1$ disease by numerous individuals. Survival results following cystectomy are similar to those attained with irradiation. Although complications and morbidity may be seen following radiotherapy, these are not as severe problems as are encountered after cystectomy and urinary diversion; the operative *mortality* alone is more than ten per cent in most institutions.

*Stage $B_2$ and C:* Perhaps 50 per cent of patients with clinical Stage $B_2$ and C bladder tumors have disease in pelvic lymph nodes. Therefore, therapy must be fashioned to include this region. Treatment of the whole pelvis with a four field technique to a dose of 5,500 rads in 5 to 5½ weeks is suggested; an additional 1,000 rads is then given to the bladder proper through small portals. These patients also must be followed closely postirradiation. Cystectomy is done, if feasible, for biopsy proven persistence three months or more following irradiation.

The results of cystectomy alone or following preoperative irradiation are no better than with radiotherapy alone. Since the morbidity is appreciably less following irradiation than following cystectomy, until further evidence is forthcoming, the available clinical data would favor radiotherapy as the primary mode of treatment.

*Stage $D_1$:* An occasional patient with Stage $D_1$ disease can be cured with external radiotherapy. The whole pelvis must be treated to doses of at least 5,500 rads, with boost therapy to the bladder and other areas of known disease.

Split-course radiotherapy may be particularly beneficial for patients with such advanced disease. Doses of 3,000 rads in 12 treatments over 2½ weeks are usually well tolerated. After a rest period of approximately 2 to 2½ weeks, the patient is re-evaluated and if there is no contraindication for further therapy, then an additional 3,000 rads are given in 10 to 12 treatments over 2 to 2½ weeks.

***Stage D₂:*** Radiotherapy is indicated for palliation only. The dose and region treated depends on the individual case.

5-fluorouracil, given intravenously, may be beneficial although the results in the literature are equivocal still in this regard. Fifteen milligrams per kilogram for five days is a common primary dose. Maintenance therapy is then individualized.

In summary, the 1935 advice of Colston and Leadbetter[55] still seems valid: "Radical surgical procedures, including total cystectomy, should be reserved for those cases which have proven resistant to a thorough course of deep x ray and radium therapy." Advances have developed with operative procedures since that time, but radiotherapy likewise is very much more effective, because of better quality radiations, more adequate knowledge of radiation physics and radiobiology, and better trained and qualified radiotherapists and ancillary personnel.

# Bibliography

1. ABBASSIAN, A., and WALLACE, D. M.: Intracavitary chemotherapy of diffuse non-infiltrating papillary carcinoma of the bladder. *J. Urol.*, 96:461-465, 1966.
2. ALLEGRA, S. R., *et al.:* Cytologic diagnosis of occult and "in-situ" carcinoma of the urinary system. *Acta Cytol.*, 10:340-349, 1966.
3. ALLEN, C. V.: Carcinoma of the urinary bladder. *Radiol. Clin.*, 33:7-12, 1964.
4. AMAR, A. D.: Bladder tumor diagnosis: Improved excretory cystograms. *Calif. Med.*, 106:120-123, 1967.
5. ASCHNER, P. W.: The pathology of vesical neoplasms: Its evaluation in diagnosis and prognosis. *J.A.M.A.*, 91:1697-1704, 1928.
6. BAKER, R.: Relation of circumferential lymphatic spread of vesical cancer with depth of infiltration: Relation to present methods of treatment. *J. Urol.*, 73:681-690, 1955.
7. BAKER, R., *et al.:* Regeneration of transitional epithelium of the human bladder after total surgical excision for recurrent, multiple bladder cancer: Apparent tumor inhibition. *J. Urol.*, 93:593-597, 1965.
8. BAKER, R.: The accuracy of clinical vs surgical staging. *J.A.M.A.*, 206:1770-1773, 1968.
9. BARNES, R. W., *et al.:* Control of bladder tumors by endoscopic surgery. *J. Urol.*, 97:864-868, 1967.
10. BARRINGER, B. S.: Radium treatment of cancer of the bladder. *Ann. Surg.*, 101:1425-1432, 1935.
11. BARRINGER, B. S.: Five-year control of bladder cancers by radon implants. *J.A.M.A.*, 120:909-911, 1942.
12. BARTLEY, O., and ECKERBOM, H.: Perivesical insufflation of gas for determination of bladder wall thickness in tumors of the bladder. *Acta Radiol.*, 54:241-248, 1960.
13. BEER, E.: Some remarks on five year cures in malignant tumors, *S. G. O.*, 60:479-480, 1935.

14. BEGG, R. C.: Colloid tumors of the urachus invading the bladder. *Brit. J. Surg.*, 23:769-772, 1936.

15. BERGKVIST, A., *et al.:* Classification of bladder tumors based on the cellular pattern: Preliminary reports of a clinical-pathological study of 300 cases with a minimum follow-up of eight years. *Acta Chir. Scand.*, 130:371-378, 1965.

16. BERMAN, H. I.: Urinary diversion in treatment of carcinoma of bladder. *Surg. Clin. N. A.*, 45:1495-1508, 1965.

17. BERRY, N. E., and WHITE, E. P.: The endoscopic treatment of bladder tumours. *Brit. J. Urol.*, 29:226-227, 1957.

18. BLOEDORN, F. G.: Carcinoma of the bladder, in *Textbook of Radiotherapy* by Fletcher, G. H. Lea & Febiger, Philadelphia, 1966, pp. 504-520.

19. BLOEDORN, F. G., *et al.:* Radiotherapy in carcinoma of the bladder: Possible complications and their prevention. *Radiology*, 79:576-581, 1962.

20. BLOEDORN, F. G., *et al.:* Radiotherapy in the treatment of cancer of the bladder. *South Med. J.*, 60:539-544, 1967.

21. BLOOM, H. J. G.: Treatment of carcinoma of the bladder: 1. Treatment by interstitial irradiation using tantalum 182 wire. *Brit. J. Radiol.*, 33:471-479, 1960.

22. BOIJSEN, E., and NILSSON, J.: Angiography in the diagnosis of tumors of the urinary bladder. *Acta Radiol.*, 57:241-258, 1962.

23. BONSER, G. M.: The experimental induction of cancer of the bladder. *Acta Unio Internat. Contra Cancerum*, 18:538-544, 1962.

24. BONSER, G. M.: Experimental studies as a background to the prevention of tumors of the urinary tract, in *The Prevention of Cancer.* Appleton-Century-Crofts, New York, 1967, pp. 237-243.

25. BOTSTEIN, C.: Four years experience with cancer of the bladder treated with high-speed electrons, in *Frontiers of Radiation Therapy and Oncology.* S. Karger Basel, New York, 1968, pp. 238-247.

26. BOWLES, W. T.: Carcinoma of the urinary bladder. *Med. Times*, 94:735-739, 1966.

27. BOWLES, W. T., and CORDONNIER, J. J.: Total cystectomy for carcinoma of the bladder. *J. Urol.*, 90:731-735, 1963.

28. BOYLAND, E.: Urinary metabolites as causative agents in bladder cancer. *Acta Unio Internat. Contra Cancerum*, 18:545-547, 1962.

29. BOYLAND, E.: Attempted prophylaxis of bladder cancer with 1→4 glucosaccharolactone. *Brit. J. Urol.*, 36:563-569, 1964.

30. BOYLAND, E., *et al.:* The induction of carcinoma of the bladder in rats with acetamidofluorene. *Brit. J. Cancer*, 8:647-654, 1954.

31. BRACK, C. B., *et al.:* Neoplasms of the female urinary bladder. *J. Urol.*, 80:24-30, 1958.

32. BRADY, L. W., and GISLASON, G. J.: The management of carcinoma of the bladder using supervoltage modalities. *Amer. J. Roentgenol.*, 89:150-154, 1963.

33. BRATHERTON, D. G.: The treatment of bladder growths by a solid intravesical cobalt source. *Brit. J. Radiol.*, 28:508-513, 1955.

34. BRICE, M., II: Radical total cystectomy for cancer of the bladder: 10 years later, in *Fifth National Cancer Conference Proceedings.* Philadelphia, Lippincott, 1964, pp. 303-307.

*one hundred and two*

35. BRICKER, E. M.: Bladder substitution after pelvic evisceration. *Surg. Clin. N. A.,* 30:1511-1521, 1966.
36. BRIZEL, H. E., and SCOTT, R. M.: Palliative irradiation for bladder carcinoma. *Amer. J. Roentgenol.,* 100:909-915, 1967.
37. BROBST, D. F., and OLSON, C.: Histopathology of urinary bladder tumors induced by bovine cutaneous papilloma agent. *Cancer Res.,* 25:12-19, 1965.
38. BRODERS, A. C.: Epithelioma of the genito-urinary organs. *Ann. Surg.,* 75: 574-580, 1922.
39. BROWNE, H. H., and OGDEN, R. T.: Rotational cobalt 60 teletherapy of vesicle cancer. *Amer. J. Roentgenol.,* 83:107-115, 1960.
40. BRUNSCHWIG, A., and BARBER, H. R. K.: Secondary and tertiary rediversion of the urinary tract, *J.A.M.A.,* 203:617-620, 1968.
41. BURNAM, C. F.: The treatment of malignant epithelial new growths of the urinary bladder. *South. Med. J.,* 26:136-144, 1933.
42. BURT, F. B., *et al.:* Heterotransplantation of bladder cancer in the hamster cheek pouch: In vivo testing of cancer chemotherapeutic agents. *J. Urol.,* 95:51-57, 1966.
43. BUSBY, S. M.: Cobalt beam therapy in primary bladder tumours: A five-year review. *Canad. J. Surg.,* 1:69-73, 1957.
44. BUSCHKE, F., and CANTRIL, S. T.: Roentgentherapy of carcinoma of urinary bladder: An analysis of 52 patients treated with 800 KV roentgentherapy. *J. Urol.,* 48:368-383, 1942.
45. BUSCHKE, F., and JACK, G.: Twenty-five years' experience with supervoltage therapy in the treatment of transitional cell carcinoma of the bladder. *Amer. J. Roentgenol.,* 99:387-392, 1967.
46. CADE, I. S., and McEWEN, J. B.: Megavoltage radiotherapy in hyperbaric oxygen. *Cancer,* 20:817-821, 1967.
47. CALDWELL, W. L.: Radiotherapy of bladder tumors. *J.A.M.A.,* 200:183, 1967.
48. CALDWELL, W. L., *et al.:* Efficacy of linear accelerator x-ray therapy in cancer of the bladder. *J. Urol.,* 97:294-303, 1967.
49. CASE, R. A. M.: Tumours of the urinary tract as an occupational disease in several industries. *Ann. Roy. Coll. Surg.,* 39:213-235, 1966.
50. CHAPMAN, T. L., and SUTHERLAND, J. W.: The clinical significance of biopsy examination of bladder tumours. *Brit. J. Urol.,* 26:369-374, 1954.
51. CHAPMAN, W. H.: Effects of oral tobacco tar and a paraffin foreign body on the mouse bladder, in *Bladder Cancer.* Aesculapius Publishing Co., Birmingham, Ala., 1967, pp. 170-178.
52. COBB, B. G., and ANSELL, J. S.: Cigarette smoking and cancer of the bladder. *J.A.M.A.,* 93:329-332, 1965.
53. COCKETT, A. T. K., *et al.:* Enhancement of regional bladder megavoltage irradiation in the bladder cancer using local bladder hyperthermia. *J. Urol.,* 97:1034-1039, 1967.
54. COLLINS, C. D.: Influence of previous surgery on results of megavoltage radiotherapy in carcinoma of bladder. *Lancet,* 2:988-990, 1964.
55. COLSTON, J. A. C., and LEADBETTER, W. F.: Infiltrating carcinoma of the bladder. *J. Urol.,* 36:669-689, 1936.
56. CONES, D. M. T., and GREGORY, C.: A technique for intracavitary radiation of the bladder. *Brit. J. Radiol.,* 25:597-600, 1952.
57. CONNOLLY, J. G., *et al.:* An evaluation of the fractionated cystogram in the

*one hundred and three*

assessment of infiltrating tumors of the bladder. *J. Urol.,* 98:356-360, 1967.

58. CORDONNIER, J. J.: Cystectomy in the management of carcinoma of the urinary bladder. *Postgrad. Med. J.,* 41:469-470, 1965.

59. CORDONNIER, J. J.: Cystectomy for carcinoma of the bladder. *J. Urol.,* 99:172-173, 1968.

60. CORDONNIER, J. J., and SEAMAN, W. B.: Betatron therapy in advanced carcinoma of the urinary bladder. *J. Urol.,* 76:256-262, 1956.

61. COX, R.: Treatment of carcinoma of the bladder II. Treatment by 2 Mev x-rays. *Brit. J. Radiol.,* 33:480-483, 1960.

62. CRIGLER, C. M., *et al.:* Radiotherapy for carcinoma of the bladder. *J. Urol.,* 96:55-61, 1966.

63. CUCCIA, C. A.: Intracavitary or interstitial use of isotopes in carcinoma of the urinary bladder. *J. Urol.,* 79:94-98, 1958.

64. DALRYMPLE, J. O.: Bladder tumours in rubber workers. *Proc. Royal Soc. Med.* 60:122-124, 1967.

65. DAMON, J. E., and WOODRUFF, M. S.: Care and management of the ureteroileostomy patient. *N. Y. State J. of Med.,* 62:3244-3247, 1962.

66. DAVIES, J. M.: Bladder tumours in electric-cable industry. *Lancet,* 2:143-146, 1965.

67. DAVIES, J. M.: Occupational bladder cancers: Epidemiology of occupational tumors of the bladder. *Proc. Royal Soc. Med.,* 59:1247-1254, 1966.

68. DEAN, A. L.: Comparison of the malignancy of bladder tumors as shown by the cystoscopic biopsy and subsequent examination of the entire excised organ. *J. Urol.,* 59:193-194, 1948.

69. DEAN, A. L., *et al.:* A restudy of the first 1,400 tumors in the bladder tumor registry, Armed Forces Institute of Pathology. *J. Urol.,* 71:571-590, 1954.

70. DEELEY, T. J., and COHEN, S. L.: The relationship between cancer of the bladder and smoking, in *Bladder Cancer.* Aesculapius Publishing Co., Birmingham, Ala., 1967, pp. 163-168.

71. DEICHMANN, W. B.: Introduction, in *Bladder Cancer,* Aesculapius Publishing Co., Birmingham, Ala., 1967, pp. 3-34.

72. DEL REGATO, J. A., and CHAHBAZIAN, C. M.: Radiotherapy for Transitional Cell Carcinoma of the Urinary Bladder with Cobalt 60. Presented at the Annual Meeting of the Radiological Society of N. A., 1966.

73. DEREN, T. L., and WILSON, W. L.: Use of 5-Fluorouracil in treatment of bladder carcinomas. *J. Urol.,* 83:390-393, 1960.

74. DE WEERD, J. H., and COLBY, M. Y.: Bladder carcinoma: Combined radiotherapy and surgical treatment. *J.A.M.A.,* 199:109-111, 1967.

75. DICK, D. A. L.: Carcinoma of the bladder treated by external irradiation. *Brit. J. Urol.,* 34:340-350, 1962.

76. DICKSON, R. J., and LANG, E. K.: Treatment of papillomata of the bladder with radioactive colloidal gold (Au[198]). *Amer. J. Roentgenol.,* 83:116-122, 1960.

77. DOLL, R.: Discussion of papers on occupational bladder cancers. *Proc. Roy. Soc. Med.,* 59:1253-1254, 1966.

78. DOYLE, F. H.: Cystography in bladder tumors: A technique using "Steripaque" and carbon dioxide. *Brit. J. Rad.,* 34:205-215, 1961.

79. DOYLE, F. H.: Bladder cancer, double contrast cystography and a bladder analogue. *Brit. J. Rad.,* 36:306-318, 1963.

*one hundred and four*

80. DRAPER, J. W., *et al.*: Vesical carcinogenesis after bladder epithelial replacement. *J. Urol.*, 97:669-678, 1967.
81. DREW, J. E., and MARSHALL, V. F.: The effects of topical thiotepa on the recurrence rate of superficial bladder cancers. *J. Urol.* 99:740-743, 1968.
82. DUCKWORTH, D. A.: The treatment of papillomatosis with podophyllin. *J. Urol.*, 64:740, 1950.
83. DURAND, L.: Endoscopic treatment of cancer of the urinary bladder, in *XIII Congres de la Societe Internationale d'Urologie*. E. and S. Livingstone, Ltd., Edinburgh & London, 1964, vol. 2, pp. 157-172.
84. EDSMYR, F., and NILSON, A. E.: Vesico-ureteric reflux in connection with supervoltage therapy for bladder carcinoma. *Acta Radiol.*, 3:449-456, 1965.
85. EDSMYR, F., *et al.*: Cobalt 60 teletherapy of carcinoma of the bladder. *Acta Radiol.*, 6:81-99, 1967.
86. EDWARDS, D. N.: Complications following megavoltage radiation for carcinoma of the bladder. *Clin. Radiol.*, 16:27-33, 1965.
87. EINHORN, H., *et al.*: Treatment of papillomatosis of the bladder with radioactive arsenic ($^{76}$As). *Acta Radiol.*, 2:1-16, 1964.
88. EISENBERG, H.: End-results in cancer of the prostate and the urinary bladder, 1940 to 1959, in *Fifth National Cancer Conference Proceedings*, Philadelphia, Lippincott, 1964, pp. 331-340.
89. ELLIS, F.: Bladder neoplasms—The challenge to the radiotherapist. *Clin. Radiol.*, 14:1-16, 1963.
90. ELLIS, F., and OLIVER, R.: Treatment of papilloma of bladder with radioactive colloidal gold (Au$^{198}$). *Brit. Med. J.*, 1:136-139, 1955.
91. EMMETT, J. L., and WINTERRINGER, J. R.: Experience with implantation of radon seeds for bladder tumors: Comparison of results with other forms of treatment. *J. Urol.*, 73:502-515, 1955.
92. ESQUIVEL, E. L., *et al.*: Treatment of bladder tumors by instillation of thiotepa, actinomycin D., or 5-fluorouracil. *Invest. Urol.*, 2:381-386, 1965.
93. FAHMY, A.: Histological grading of urinary bladder tumours. *Urol. Int.* 15: 358-377, 1963.
94. FARRELL, J. T., and FETTER, T. R.: Roentgen irradiation in carcinoma of the bladder: A series of 72 cases. *J. Urol.*, 37:133-140, 1937.
95. FERGUSON, R. S.: Results of treatment of the genito-urinary tumors by roentgen rays. *J. Urol.*, 37:823-831, 1937.
96. FINNEY, R.: The treatment of carcinoma of the bladder with megavoltage irradiation—A clinical trial. *Clin. Radiol.*, 16:324-327, 1965.
97. FINNEY, R.: Personal Communication, 1967.
98. FINNEY, R., and JONES, H. C.: Megavoltage therapy in carcinoma of the bladder. *Lancet*, 1:580-582, 1962.
99. FLOCKS, R. H.: Treatment of Patients with Carcinoma of the Bladder. *J.A.M.A.* 145:295-301, 1951.
100. FRANK, H. G.: The radiological assessment of bladder tumors: Part 2. Radiotherapy. *J. Urol.*, 92:484-489, 1964.
101. FRANKSSON, C.: Tumors of the urinary bladder. *Acta Chir. Scand.*, 100 (Suppl. 151): 1-203, 1950.
102. FRAUMENI, J. F., JR.: Cigarette smoking and cancers of the urinary tract: Geographic variations in the United States. *J. Nat. Cancer Inst.*, 41:1205-1211, 1968.

*one hundred and five*

103. FRAUMENI, J. F., JR., and THOMAS, L. B.: Malignant bladder tumors in a man and his three sons. *J.A.M.A.*, 201:507-509, 1967.

104. FRIEDELL, G. H., and BURNEY, S. W.: Bladder cancer: An increasing problem. *Cancer Bull.*, 20:42-45, May-June, 1968.

105. FRIEDDELL, G. H., and McAULEY, R. L.: Untreated bladder cancer: 31 autopsy cases. *J. Urol.*, 100:293-296, 1968.

106. FRIEDMAN, M.: Supervoltage (2 mvp) rotation irradiation of cancer of the bladder. *Radiology*, 73:191-208, 1959.

107. FRIEDMAN, M.: Radioisotope techniques: Intracavity placement of radium, interstitial implantations, and instillations. *J.A.M.A.*, 206:2722-2723, 1968.

108. FRIEDMAN, M., and LEWIS, L. G.: A new technic for the radium treatment. *Radiology*, 53:342-363, 1949.

109. FRIEDMAN, M., and LEWIS, L. G.: Irradiation of carcinoma of the bladder by a central intracavitary radium or cobalt 60 source (The Walter Reed Technique). *Amer. J. Roentgenol.*, 79:6-31,1958.

110. FRIEDMAN, N. B., and ASH, J. E.: *Tumors of the Urinary Bladder.* Armed Forces Institute of Pathology, Washington, D. C., 1959.

111. GALLEHER, E. P., *et al.*: A followup study of supervoltage irradiation followed by cystectomy for bladder cancer. *J. Urol.*, 99:59-64, 1968.

112. GALLEHER, E. P., *et al.*: Supervoltage irradiation followed by cystectomy for bladder cancer. *J. Urol.*, 93:598-603, 1965.

113. GELFAND, M., *et al.*: Relation between carcinoma of the bladder and infestation with Schistosoma Haematobium. *Lancet*, 1:1249-1251, 1967.

114. GLANTZ, G. M.: Cystectomy and urinary diversion, *J. Urol.*, 96:714-717, 1966.

115. GLANVILLE, J. N.: The radiological assessment of bladder tumors: Part I. Radiodiagnosis. *J. Urol.*, 5:479-483, 1964.

116. GOLDSTEIN, A. G., *et al.*: Haemorrhagic radiation cystitis. *Brit. J. Urol.*, 40: 475-478, 1968.

117. GOODMAN, G. B., and BALFOUR, J.: Carcinoma of bladder: Cobalt therapy. *J. Urol.*, 92:30-36, 1964.

118. GOODMAN, G. B., and BALFOUR, J.: Local recurrence of bladder cancer after supervoltage irradiation. *J. Canad. Assoc. Radiol.*, 15:92-98, 1964.

119. GOWING, N. F. C.: Urethral carcinoma associated with cancer of bladder. *Brit. J. Urol.*, 32:428-439, 1960.

120. GRABSTALD, H.: *In situ* and invasive carcinoma of the urinary bladder, in *Bladder Cancer.* Aesculapius Publishing Co., Birmingham, Ala., 1967, pp. 207-210.

121. GRACE, D. A., and WINTER, C. C.: Mixed differentiation of primary carcinoma of the urinary bladder. *Cancer*, 21:1239-1243, 1968.

122. GREENSLADE, N. F., *et al.*: Tumours of the bladder in Canterbury, New Zealand: A study of incidence and results of treatment, 1953-62. *Brit. J. Surg.*, 52:841-846, 1965.

123. GUTTMAN, R., and BAUZA, A.: The treatment of advanced carcinoma of the bladder. *Radiology*, 77:465-471, 1961.

124. HANLEY, H. G.: The rectal bladder. *Brit. J. Surg.*, 53:678-681, 1966.

125. HARADA, N., and KUSUNOKI, T.: Results of the mucosal denudation for bladder tumors: An interim report. *J. Urol.*, 99:725-732, 1968.

126. HARRIS, W.: Discussion of paper by Friedman, M. and Lewis, L. G.: Radium treatment of carcinoma of bladder. *Radiology*, 53:361-362, 1949.

*one hundred and six*

127. Hecker, G. N., et al.: Radical cystectomy after supervoltage radiotherapy, J. Urol., 91:256-260, 1964.

128. Herring, H. T.: The treatment of vesical papilloma by injections. Brit. Med. J., 2:1398, 1903.

129. Higgins, P. M., et al.: The hazards of total cystectomy after supervoltage irradiation of the bladder. Brit. J. Urol., 38:311-318, 1966.

130. Hinman, F., et al.: Further experience with intracavitary radiocobalt for bladder tumors. J. Urol., 73:285-291, 1955.

131. Hodt, H. J., et al.: Gun for interstitial implantation of radioactive gold grains. Brit. J. Radiol., 25:419-421, 1952.

132. Holsti, L. R., and Ermala, P.: Papillary carcinoma of the bladder in mice, obtained after perioral administration of tobacco tar, Cancer 8:679-682, 1955.

133. Holsti, L. R.: Split-course radiotherapy of cancer. Acta Radiol., 6:313-322, 1967.

134. Hueper, W. C.: Environmental and industrial cancers of the urinary bladder in the U. S. A. Acta Unio Internat. Contra Cancerum, 18:585-596, 1962.

135. Hueper, W. C., Wiley, F. H., and Wolfe, H. D.: Experimenal production of bladder tumors in dogs by administration of beta-naphthylamine. J. Ind. Hyg. Toxicol., 20:46-84, 1938.

136. Immergut, M.: Carcinoma of the bladder: A death associated with the toxicity of combined therapy with 5-fluorouracil and cobalt irradiation. J. Urol., 99:169-171, 1968.

137. Jack, G., and Buschke, F.: The role of external irradiation in the treatment of transitional cell carcinoma of the bladder: A review of fifty cases. Calif. Med., 106:12-16, 1967.

138. Jacobs, A.: Carcinoma of the bladder, 1. The treatment of cancer of the bladder by radium. Brit. J. Radiol., 22:393-408, 1949.

139. Jewett, H. J.: Carcinoma of the bladder: Influence of depth of infiltration on the 5-year results following complete extirpation of the primary growth. J. Urol., 67:672-680, 1952.

140. Jewett, H. J.: Carcinoma of the bladder: Development and evaluation of current concepts of therapy. J. Urol., 82:92-100, 1959.

141. Jewett, H. J.: Prognosis of bladder tumors based on anatomical and pathological study, in XIII Congres de la Societe Internationale d'Urologie. E. and S. Livingstone, Ltd., Edinburgh & London, 1:138-154, 1964.

142. Jewett, H. J.: Conservative treatment vs radical surgery for superficial cancer of the bladder. J.A.M.A., 206:2720-2721, 1968.

143. Jewett, H. J., and Eversole, S. L.: Carcinoma of the bladder: Characteristic modes of local invasion. J. Urol., 83:383-389, 1960.

144. Jewett, H. J., and Strong, G. H.: Infiltrating carcinoma of the bladder: Relation of depth of penetration of the bladder wall to incidence of local extension and metastases. J. Urol., 55:366-372, 1946.

145. Jewett, H. J., et al.: A study of 365 cases of infiltrating bladder cancer: Relationship of certain pathological characteristics to prognosis after extirpation. J. Urol., 92:668-678, 1964.

146. Jones, H. C., and Swinney, J.: ThioTepa in the treatment of tumours of the bladder. Lancet, 2:615-618, 1961.

147. Kaufman, J. J.: The management of tumours of the bladder. Practitioner, 197:611-619, 1966.

*one hundred and seven*

148. KAUFMAN, J. J.: Cancer of the bladder—Experiences using combined chemotherapy, radiotherapy, and surgery. Presented at Third Annual Radiotherapy Symposium on Current Concepts in Diagnosis and Management of Genitourinary Tumors, Miami, January 23-25, 1969.

149. KAUFMAN, J. J., and LICHTENAUR, P.: Cancer of human bladder: Responses of tumor xenografts to chemotherapy and radiotherapy. *Cancer,* 21:1-8, 1968.

150. KAUFMAN, J. J., and STEIN, J. J.: 5-Fluorouracil (NSC-19893) combined with cobalt 60 teletherapy in treatment of bladder cancer—preliminary report. *Cancer Chemother. Rep.,* No. 48:65-71, 1965.

151. KAUFMAN, H., *et al.:* Findings on angiography of the pelvis in carcinoma of the bladder. *Fortschr. a. d. Geb. d. Roentgenstrahlen,* 105:802-806, 1966.

152. KERN, W. H., *et al.:* Cytologic evaluation of the transitional cell carcinoma of the bladder. *J. Urol.,* 100:616-622, 1968.

153. KERR, W. K., *et al.:* A hypernephroma associated with elevated levels of bladder carcinogens in the urine: Case report. *Brit. J. Urol.,* 35:263-266, 1963.

154. KING, H., and BAILAR, J. C.: Epidemiology of urinary bladder cancer. *J. Chron. Dis.,* 19:735-772, 1966.

155. KOEHLER, P. R., and BOWLES, W. T.: Radiologic evaluation of the upper urinary tract following illeal loop urinary diversion. *Radiology,* 86:227-234, 1966.

156. KUROHARA, S. S.: The forces of mortality in bladder carcinoma. *J.A.M.A.,* 207:1136-1137, 1969.

157. KUROHARA, S. S., *et al.:* Analysis in depth of bladder cancer treated by supervoltage therapy. *Amer. J. Roengenol.,* 95:458-467, 1965.

158. LAING, A. H., and DICKINSON, K. M.: Carcinoma of bladder treated by supervoltage irradiation. *Clin. Radiol.,* 16:154-164, 1965.

159. LAMB, D.: Correlation of chromosome counts with histological appearances and prognosis in transitional-cell carcinoma of bladder, *Brit. Med. J.,* 1:273-277, 1967.

160. LANG, E. K.: Use of arteriography in the demonstration and staging of bladder tumors. *Radiology,* 80:62-68, 1963.

161. LANG, E. K.: Triple cystogram and selective arteriography. *J.A.M.A.,* 207: 342-344, 1969.

162. LANG, E. K., *et al.:* Retrograde arteriography in the staging and follow-up bladder tumors. *Radiology,* 80:267-269, 1963.

163. LASKOWSKI, T. Z., *et al.:* Combined therapy: Radiation and surgery in the treatment of bladder cancer, *J. Urol.,* 99:733-739, 1968.

164. Leading Article: Radical bladder surgery. *Brit. Med. J.,* 1:188, 1967.

165. Leading Article: Early diagnosis of bladder cancer. *Brit. Med. J.,* 1:253-254, 1967.

166. LEIGNER, L. M., *et al.:* Supervoltage cobalt-60 treatment of bladder cancer: Palliation or cure? *J. Urol.,* 87:373-380, 1962.

167. LENZ, M., *et al.:* The treatment of cancer of the bladder by radium needles. *Amer. J. Roentgenol.,* 58:486-492, 1947.

168. LEROI, A., and LEROI-VON MAY (ARLESHEIM): Handling of malignant bladder tumors with mistletoe extract. *Zschr. Urol.,* 51:555, 1958.

169. LEVIN, J., *et al.:* An appraisal of renal function and infection in advanced bladder cancer treated with ileal bladder construction and irradiation. *S. G. O.,* 112:53-60, 1961.

*one hundred and eight*

170. Lockwood, K.: On the etiology of bladder tumors in Kobenhavn-Frederiksberg. *Acta Unio Internat. Contra Cancerum,* 18:608-610, 1962.

171. Lougheed, M. N.: Principles of radiation therapy in bladder tumours. *Brit. J. Urol.,* 29:236-240, 1957.

172. MacKay, N. R.: Tolerance of the bladder to intracavitary irradiation. *J. Urol.,* 76:396-400, 1956.

173. MacKenzie, A. R., and Whitmore, W. F. Jr.: Resection of pubic rami for urologic cancer. *J. Urol.,* 100:546-551, 1968.

174. MacKenzie, A. R., *et al.:* Supervoltage x-ray therapy of bladder cancer. *Cancer,* 18:1255-1260, 1965.

175. MacKenzie, A. R., *et al.:* Myosarcomas of the bladder and prostate. *Cancer,* 22:833-844, 1968.

176. McDonald, J. R., and Thompson, G. J.: Carcinoma of the urinary bladder: A pathologic study with special reference to invasiveness and vascular invasion. *J. Urol.,* 60:435-445, 1948.

177. McEwen, J. B.: Clinical trial of radiotherapy and high pressure oxygen. *Ann. Roy. Coll. Surg.,* 39:168-171, 1966.

178. McLean, P., and Kelalis, P. P.: Bladder diverticulum in the male. *Brit. J. Urol.,* 40:321-323, 1968.

179. Magri, J.: Partial cystectomy: A review of 104 cases. *Brit. J. Urol.,* 34:74-87, 1962.

180. Makar, N.: Some observations on pseudo-glandular proliferations in the bilharzial bladder, *Acta Unio Internat. Contra Cancerum,* 18:599-610, 1962.

181. Malignant Tumors of the Urinary Bladder: Clinical Stage Classification and Presentation of Results. Subcommittee of Clinical Stage Classification and Applied Statistics, Geneva. Union Internationale Centre le Cancerum, 1967, pp. 3-17.

182. Maltry, E.: Carcinoma of the bladder, *J. Urol.,* 99:165-168, 1968.

183. Mancuso, T. F., and El-Attar, A. A.: Cohort study of workers exposed to betanaphthylamine and benzidine. *J. Occup. Med.,* 9:277-285, 1967.

184. Marshall, V. F.: The relation of the preoperative estimate to the pathologic demonstration of the extent of vesical neoplasms. *J. Urol.,* 68:714-723. 1952.

185. Marshall, V. F.: Current clinical problems regarding bladder tumors. *Cancer,* 9:543-550, 1956.

186. Marshall, V. F.: The choice of surgical therapy for epithelial neoplasms of the urinary Bladder, *Brit. J. Urol.,* 29:228-231, 1957.

187. Marshall, V. F.: *Textbook of Urology,* 2nd Ed. New York, Evanston, London, Hoeber, 1964.

188. Marshall, V. F., *et al.:* Survival of patients with bladder carcinoma treated by simple segmental resection. *Cancer,* 9:568-571, 1956.

189. Masina, F.: Segmental resection for tumours of the urinary bladder: Ten-year follow-up. *Brit. J. Surg.,* 52:279-283, 1965.

190. Masuda, Y., *et al.:* Studies on bladder carcinogens in the human environment I. Naphthylamines produced by pyrolysis of amino acids. *Int. J. Cancer,* 2:489-493, 1967.

191. Mechl, Z., *et al.:* Tentative treatment of bladder tumors by a combination of instillation of thio-tepa followed by irradiation. *Cesko. Radiol.,* 20:21-24, 1966.

*one hundred and nine*

192. MELAMED, M. R.: Clinicopathologic features of carcinogenesis in the human urinary bladder, in *Bladder Cancer*. Aesculapius Publishing Co., Birmingham, Ala., 1967, pp. 200-206.

193. MELAMED, M. R., *et al.*: Natural history and clinical behavior of *in situ* carcinoma of the human urinary bladder. *Cancer*, 17:1533-1545, 1964.

194. MELAMED, M. R., *et al.*: Carcinoma *in situ* of bladder: Clinico-pathologic study of case with a suggested approach to detection. *J. Urol.*, 96:466-471, 1966.

195. MELICK, W. F., and NARYKA, J. J.: Carcinoma *in situ* of the bladder in workers exposed to xenylamine: Diagnosis by ultraviolet light cystoscopy. *J. Urol.*, 99:178-182, 1968.

196. MELICOW, M. M.: Tumors of the urinary bladder: A clinicopathological analysis of over 2500 specimens and biopsies. *J. Urol.*, 74:498-521, 1955.

197. MILLEN, J. L. E.: Carcinoma of the bladder, III. Treatment by radon seed implantation and deep x-ray therapy. *Brit. J. Radiol.*, 22:402-405, 1949.

198. MILLER, L. S., *et al.*: Supervoltage irradiation for carcinoma of the urinary bladder. *Radiol.*, 82:778-784, 1964.

199. MILNER, W. A.: Transurethral biopsy: An accurate method of determining the true malignancy of bladder carcinoma. *J. Urol.*, 61:917-929, 1949.

200. MILNER, W. A.: End results in the treatment of bladder tumors. *J. Urol.*, 69:657-664, 1953.

201. MILNER, W. A.: The role of conservative surgery in the treatment of bladder tumours. *Brit. J. Urol.*, 27:375-386, 1955.

202. MOORE, V., *et al.*: Experiences with radioactive chromic phosphate in urological tumours. *Arch. Surg.*, 72:464-468, 1956.

203. MORRISON, R., and DEELEY, T. J.: The treatment of recurrent carcinoma of the bladder by supervoltage radiotherapy. *Brit. J. Urol.*, 38:319-322, 1966.

204. MORRISON, R., *et al.*: The treatment of carcinoma of the bladder by supervoltage x-rays. *Brit. J. Radiol.*, 38:449-458, 1965.

205. Moss, W. T.: *Therapeutic Radiology*, 3rd Ed., C. V. Mosby Company, St. Louis, 1969, pp. 314-327.

206. MOSTOFI, R. K.: Pathology of cancer of bladder. *Acta Unio Internat. Contra Cancerum*, 18:611-615, 1962.

207. MOSTOFI, F. K.: Pathological aspects and spread of carcinoma of the bladder. *J.A.M.A.*, 206:1764-1769, 1968.

208. MOUSA, A. H.: Bilharziasis and prevention of bladder cancer in Egypt, in *The Prevention of Cancer*. Appleton-Century-Crofts, New York, 1967, pp. 253-256.

209. MULLER, J. H.: Radiotherapy of bladder cancer by means of rubber balloons filled *in situ* with solutions of a radioactive isotope ($Co^{60}$). *Cancer*, 8: 1035-1042, 1955.

210. NEWMAN, D. M., *et al.*: Squamous cell carcinoma of the bladder. *J. Urol.*, 100:470-473, 1968.

211. NICHOLS, J. A., and MARSHALL, V. F.: The treatment of bladder carcinoma. *Cancer*, 9:559-565, 1956.

212. NICHOLS, J. A., and MARSHALL, V. F.: Treatment of histologically benign papilloma of the urinary bladder by local excision and fulguration. *Cancer*, 9:566-567, 1956.

213. NILSSON, J.: Angiography in tumours of the urinary bladder. *Acta Radiol.*, Suppl. 263, 1967.

*one hundred and ten*

214. Oppenheimer, R.: The urinary tract diseases as observed by the workers in chemical firms, *Ztschr. Urol. Chir. U. Gynaek.,* 21:336-370, 1927.

215. Paces, V., *et al.:* Treatment of bladder tumors by implantation of radioactive gold grains. *Cesko. Radiol.,* 20:25-27, 1966.

216. Pamukcu, A. M., *et al.:* Urinary bladder neoplasms induced by feeding bracken fern (Pteris aquilina) to cows. *Cancer Research,* 27:917-924, 1967.

217. Paterson, R., and Pointon, R. S.: The bladder, in *The Treatment of Malignant Disease by Radiotherapy,* by Paterson, R. The Williams & Wilkins Company, Baltimore, 1963, pp. 367-383.

218. Pfahler, G. E., and Vastine, J. H.: The roengent diagnosis and treatment of tumors of the bladder: Their serial study with pneumocystograms, showing results of treatment by irradiation. *J.A.M.A.,* 104:609-613, 1935.

219. Plank, L. E., *et al.:* Cobalt-60 teletherapy for urinary bladder carcinoma: Two and one-half years' experience. *J. Urol.,* 78:402-409, 1967.

220. Pointon, R. C. S.: Bladder carcinoma. *Proc. Roy. Soc. Med.,* 53:244-246, 1960.

221. Poole-Wilson, D. S.: Surgery and irradiation in the treatment of bladder cancer. *Brit. J. Urol.,* 29:244-250, 1957.

222. Price, J. M.: Bladder cancer. *Canad. Cancer Conf.,* 6:224-243, 1966.

223. Priestley, J. T.: General considerations in the surgical treatment of carcinoma of the bladder with particular reference to total cystectomy. *N. Y. State J. Med.,* 40:1441-1449, 1940.

224. Prout, G. R.: A plan for the rational treatment of carcinoma of the bladder. *South. Med. J.,* 52:570-575, 1959.

225. Prout, G. R.: Adjuvants in the surgical treatment of bladder carcinoma, in *Cancer Therapy by Integrated Radiation and Operation.* Charles C Thomas, Springfield, Ill., 1968, pp. 119-127.

226. Prout, G. R., and Marshall, V. F.: The prognosis with untreated bladder tumors. *Cancer,* 9:551-558, 1955.

227. Prout, G. R., Jr., *et al.:* Carcinoma of the bladder, 5-Fluorouracil and the critical role of a placebo. *Cancer,* 22:926-931, 1968.

228. Pugh, R. C. B.: The grading and staging of bladder tumours. *Brit. J. Urol.,* 28:222-225, 1957.

229. Radomski, J. L., *et al.:* The metabolism of 2-naphthylamine as related to bladder carcinogenesis, in *Bladder Cancer.* Aesculapius Publishing Co., Birmingham, Ala., 1967, pp. 80-88.

230. Registry of the American Urological Association: Grading of epithelial tumors of the urinary bladder. *J. Urol.,* 36:651-668, 1963.

231. Rehn, L.: Blassengesch wulste bei Fuchsin-Arbeitern. *Arch. Klin. Chir.,* 50: 588-600, 1895.

232. Riches, E. W.: Symposium: Carcinoma of the bladder, II. Some further aspects of treatment. *Brit. J. Radiol.,* 22:398-402, 1949.

233. Riches, E. W.: Carcinoma of the bladder: The place of total cystectomy. *Brit. J. Urol.,* 29:232-235, 1957.

234. Riches, S. E.: Surgery and radiotherapy in urology: The bladder. *J. Urol.,* 90:339-350, 1963.

235. Royce, R. K., and Ackerman, L. V.: Carcinoma of the bladder: Clinical therapeutic and pathologic aspects of 135 cases. *J. Urol.,* 65:66-85, 1951.

236. Rubin, P.: The impact of supervoltage irradiation on the treatment of bladder carcinoma. *J. Urol.,* 86:82-88, 1961.

237. Saffiotti, U., et al.: Induction of bladder cancer in hamsters fed aromatic amines, in *Bladder Cancer*. Aesculapius Publishing Co., Birmingham, Ala., 1967, pp. 129-134.

238. Sagerman, R. H., et al.: Linear accelerator supervoltage radiation therapy: Carcinoma of the bladder. *Amer. J. Roentgenol.*, 93:122-127, 1965.

239. Sagerman, R. H., et al.: Preoperative irradiation for carcinoma of the bladder. *Amer. J. Roentgenol.*, 102:577-580, 1968.

240. Sambrook, D. K.: Split-course radiation therapy in malignant tumors. *Amer. J. Roentgenol.*, 91:37-45, 1964.

241. Sauer, H. R., et al.: A study of untreated bladder cancers. *J. Urol.*, 63:124-127, 1950.

242. Scanlon, P. W.: Radiotherapeutic problems best handled with split-dose therapy. *Amer. J. Roentgenol.* 93:639-650, 1965.

243. Schade, R. O. K., and Swinney, J.: Pre-cancerous changes in bladder epithelium. *Lancet*, 2:943-946, 1968.

244. Schinz, H. R.: The TNM-system of the most important cancer localization (an extract of the report of the ICPR at the IX International Congress of Radiology). *Fortschr. Rontg.*, 91:550-551, 1959.

245. Schwartz, J. W., et al.: Total cystectomy: Analysis of 225 cases from the bladder tumor registry. *J. Urol.*, 78:41-53, 1957.

246. Scott, T. S.: Occupational bladder cancers: Environmental and biological control. *Proc. Royal Soc. Med.*, 59:1248-1251, 1966.

247. Scott, W. W., and Boyd, H. L.: Study of carcinogenic effect of beta-naphthylamine of normal and substituted isolated sigmoid loop bladder of dogs, *J. Urol.*, 70:914-925, 1953.

248. Sell, A.: Intracavitary radium therapy of bladder tumours. *Danish Med. Bull.*, 14:21-26, 1967.

249. Semple, J. E.: Papillomata of the bladder treated with podophyllin. *Brit. Med. J.*, 1:1235, 1948.

250. Siegel, W. H., and Pincus, M. B.: Epithelial bladder tumors in children. *J. Urol.*, 101:55-56, 1969.

251. Simon, W., et al.: The pathogenesis of bladder carcinoma. *J. Urol.*, 88:797-802, 1962.

252. Stalport, J.: A proposed combined treatment, surgical and radiotherapy, of bladder tumors. *Acta Chir. Belg.*, 1:39-56, 1966.

253. Stein, J. J., and Kaufman, J. J.: The treatment of carcinoma of the bladder with special reference to the use of preoperative radiation therapy combined with 5-fluorouracil. *Amer. J. Roentgenol.*, 102:519-529, 1968.

254. Stitt, R. B., and Colapinto, V.: Multiple simultaneous bladder malignancies: primary lymphosarcoma and adenocarcinoma. *J. Urol.*, 96:733-736, 1966.

255. Stone, J. H., and Hodges, C. V.: Radical cystectomy for invasive bladder cancer. *J. Urol.*, 96:207-209, 1966.

256. Swinney, J.: Treatment of bladder cancer by megavoltage therapy. *Brit. J. Urol.*, 29:241-243, 1957.

257. Symanski, H. J.: The incidence of occupational cancer in the federal republic of Germany, in *Bladder Cancer*. Aesculapius Publishing Co., Birmingham, Ala., 1967, pp. 194-198.

258. Taylor, D. A., et al.: A preliminary report of a new method for the staging of bladder carcinoma using a triple contrast technique. *Brit. J. Radiol.*, 38:667-672, 1965.

*one hundred and twelve*

259. THOMPSON, G. J., and KAPLAN, J. H.: Advantages of transurethral removal of certain bladder tumors. *J. Urol.*, 73:270-279, 1955.

260. THOMPSON, N.: Carcinoma of the bladder. *Brit. J. Urol.*, 87:287-297, 1962.

261. TOMATIS, L., *et al.*: Urinary bladder and liver cell tumors induced in masters with O-aminoazotoluens. *Cancer Res.*, 21:1513-1517, 1961.

262. TSUJI, I., *et al.*: Clinical experiences of bladder reconstruction using preserved bladder and gelatin sponge bladder in the case of bladder cancer. *J. Urol.*, 98:91-92, 1967.

263. TUOVINEN, P. I., and KETTUNEN, K.: Superficial malignant lesion bladder treated by radioactive colloidal Gold ($^{198}$Au). *Brit. Med. J.* 1:1090-1092, 1967.

264. UMIKER, W.: Accuracy of cytologic diagnosis of cancer of the urinary tract. *Acta Cytol.*, 8:186-93, 1964.

265. VAN MIERT, P. J., and FOWLER, J. F.: The use of tantalum 182 in the treatment of early bladder carcinoma. *Brit. J. Radiol.*, 29:508-512, 1956.

266. VEENEMA, R. J.: The role of ThioTEPA instillations in bladder cancer. *J.A.M.A.*, 206:2725-2726, 1968.

267. VEENEMA, R. J., *et al.*: Bladder carcinoma treated by direct instillation of Thio-Tepa. *J. Urol.*, 88:60-63, 1962.

268. VEENEMA, R. J., *et al.*: Histochemistry: A possible guide to therapy of bladder tumors. *J. Urol.*, 90:736-746, 1963.

269. VEENEMA, R. J., *et al.*: Chemotherapy in bladder carcinoma, in *Fifth National Cancer Conference Proceedings*. Philadelphia, Lippincott, 1964, pp. 295-301.

270. VEENEMA, R. J., *et al.*: Combined radiotherapy, surgery and chemotherapy in carcinoma of the bladder. *Cancer*, 20:1879-1885, 1967.

271. VERMOOTEN, V., and MAXFIELD, J. G. S.: The use of radioactive cobalt in Nylon sutures in the treatment of bladder tumors technique and case reports. *J. Urol.*, 74:767-776, 1955.

272. WALINDER, G.: Colloidal $^{76}$As$_2$S$_3$: Its production and possible use in the treatment of papillomatosis of the urinary bladder. *Acta Radiol.*, 44:521-525, 1955.

273. WALLACE, D. M.: The natural history and possible cause of bladder tumours. *Ann. Roy. Coll. Surg.*, 18:366-383, 1956.

274. WALLACE, D. M.: *Tumours of Bladder*. Edinburgh and London, E.&S. Livingston, Ltd., 1959.

275. WALLACE, D. M.: Treatment of carcinoma of the bladder: 4. Surgery in the treatment of bladder tumours. *Brit. J. Radiol.*, 33:487-490, 1960.

276. WALLACE, D. M.: Occupational bladder cancers: Clinical aspects of industrial bladder tumours. *Proc. Royal Soc. Med.*, 59:1251-1254, 1966.

277. WALLACE, D. M.: Factors influencing the prognosis of early cancer of the bladder. *Proc. Royal Soc. Med.*, 59:609-610, 1966.

278. WALLACE, D. M.: The management of cancer of the bladder. *Practitioner*, 196:65-68, 1966.

279. WALLACE, D. C.: Ureteric diversion using a conduit: A simplified technique. *Brit. J. Urol.*, 38:522-527, 1966.

280. WALLACE, D. M., and HARRIS, D. L.: Delay in treating bladder tumours. *Lancet*, 2:332-334, 1965.

281. WALLACE, D. M., *et al.*: Radioactive tantalum wire implantation as a method of treatment for early carcinoma of the bladder. *Brit. J. Radiol.*, 25:421-424, 1952.

*one hundred and thirteen*

282. WALTON, R. J., and SINCLAIR, W. K.: Radioactive solutions ($^{24}$Na and $^{82}$Br) in the treatment of carcinoma of the bladder. *Brit. Med. Bull.*, 8:158-165, 1952.

283. WATSON, T. A., and CAMPBELL, J. M.: Supervoltage radiation therapy in advanced cancer of the urinary bladder. *J. Canad. Assoc. Radiol.*, 14:4-9, 1963.

284. WERF-MESSING, B. VAN DER: Telecobalt treatment of carcinoma of the bladder. *Clin. Radiol.*, 16:165-172, 1965.

285. WERF-MESSING, B. VAN DER: Treatment of carcinoma of the bladder with radium. *Clin. Radiol.*, 16:16-26, 1965.

286. WESCOTT, J. W.: The prophylactic use of Thio-Tepa in transitional cell carcinoma of the bladder. *J. Urol.*, 96:913-918, 1966.

287. WHITMORE, W. F., JR.: Preoperative irradiation combined with cystectomy in the treatment of bladder cancer, in *Fifth National Cancer Conference Proceedings*. Philadelphia, Lippincott, 1964, pp. 481-484.

288. WHITMORE, W. F., JR.: Integrated therapy for bladder cancer, in *Cancer Therapy by Integrated Radiation and Operation*, by Rush, B. F., and Greenlaw, R. H. Charles C Thomas, Springfield, Ill., 1968, pp. 111-117.

289. WHITMORE, W. F., JR., and BUSH, I. M.: Ultraviolet cystoscopy in patients with bladder cancer. *J. Urol.*, 95:201-207, 1966.

290. WHITMORE, W. F., JR., and MARSHALL, V. F.: Radical total cystectomy for cancer of the bladder: 230 consecutive cases five years later. *J. Urol.*, 87:853-868, 1962.

291. WHITMORE, W. F., JR., et al.: Experience with preoperative irradiation followed by radical cystectomy for the treatment of bladder cancer. *Amer. J. Roentgenol.*, 90:1016-1022, 1963.

292. WHITMORE, W. F. JR., et al.: Tetracycline ultraviolet fluorescence in bladder carcinoma. *Cancer*, 17:1528-1532, 1964.

293. WHITMORE, W. F., JR., et al.: Preoperative irradiation with cystectomy in the management of the bladder cancer. *Amer. J. Roentgenol.*, 102:570-576, 1968.

294. WHITMORE, W. F., JR.: Bladder cancer: Combined radiotherapy and surgical treatment. *J.A.M.A.*, 207:349-350, 1969.

295. WISE, H. M., and FAINSINGER, M. H.: Angiography in the evaluation of carcinoma of the bladder. *J.A.M.A.*, 192:1027-1031, 1965.

296. WIZENBERG, M. J., et al.: Radiation therapy and surgery in the treatment of carcinoma of the bladder. *Amer. J. Roentgenol.*, 96:113-118, 1966.

297. WOODRUFF, M. W., and MARTIN, L. S. J.: Cutaneous ileuoureterostomy: Initial clinical results in four patients. *J. Urol.*, 94:238-242, 1965.

298. WOODRUFF, M. W., et al.: Further observations on the use of combination 5-fluorouracil and supervoltage irradiation therapy in the treatment of advanced carcinoma of the bladder. *J. Urol.*, 90:747-758, 1963.

299. WYNDER, E. L., et al.: An epidemiological investigation of cancer of the bladder. *Cancer*, 16:1388-1407, 1963.

300. YOSHIDA, O.: Studies on carcinoma of the urinary bladder: 1. Statistical and epidemiological studies on cancer of the bladder in the Japanese. *Acta Urol.*, 12:1040-1064, 1966.

301. ZINSSER, H. H., et al.: Intracavitary irradiation of the bladder with radioactive B-emitting rubber balloon catheters. *Radiology*, 84:428-435, 1965.

302. ZUPPINGER, A.: The radiotherapeutic treatment of cancer of the bladder. *Min. Urol.*, 17:98-102, 1965.

*one hundred and fourteen*

# Index